Applying Evidence-Based Laboratory Medicine

Applying Evidence-Based Laboratory Medicine

A Step-by-Step Guide

Christopher P. Price, Ph.D., FRCPath, FACB
Visiting Professor in Clinical Biochemistry
University of Oxford
Oxford, UK

Joanne Lozar Glenn, M.S. Ed.
Independent Writer, Editor, Educator
Alexandria, VA
USA

Robert H. Christenson, Ph.D., DABCC, FACB
Professor of Pathology
Professor of Medical and Research Technology
University of Maryland School of Medicine
and Director, Rapid Response Laboratories
University of Maryland Medical Center
Baltimore, MD
USA

AACC Press
1850 K Street, NW, Suite 625
Washington, DC 20006

1 2 3 4 5 6 7 8 9 0 PCP 11 10 09

Printed in the United States of America

Library of Congress Cataloging-in-Publication Data

Price, Christopher P.
Applying evidence-based laboratory medicine : a step-by-step guide / Christopher P. Price, Joanne Lozar Glenn, Robert H. Christenson.
p. ; cm.
Includes bibliographical references and index.
ISBN 978-1-59425-089-7
1. Diagnosis, Laboratory--Handbooks, manuals, etc. 2. Evidence-based medicine--Handbooks, manuals, etc. I. Glenn, Joanne Lozar. II. Christenson, Robert H. III. American Association for Clinical Chemistry. IV. Title.
[DNLM: 1. Clinical Laboratory Techniques--methods--Handbooks. 2. Decision Making--Handbooks. 3. Evidence-Based Medicine--methods--Handbooks. QY 39 P9455a 2008]

RB38.2.P78 2008
616.07'5--dc22

2008022355

To Lucy
—CPP

To my coauthors—your spirit of collaboration and inquiry, and your flexibility of mind, are outstanding and much admired. To Joanna Grimes—your dedication and attention to detail are unparalleled and also much admired.
—JLG

To Karen and Lloyd Anderson. You are incredibly kind.
—RHC

CONTENTS

Foreword viii

Preface x

About This Book: What to Expect and How to Use It xiv

Part 1: An Introduction to Evidence-Based Laboratory Medicine 1

Part 2: Steps in EBLM—The A5 Cycle 43

Step A1: ASK—Formulate an Answerable Question 43

Step A2: ACQUIRE—Find the Evidence 89

Step A3: APPRAISE—Critically Evaluate the Evidence 117

Step A4: APPLY—Apply the Evidence to Your Clinical Situation 147

Step A5: ASSESS—Audit the Process 175

Part 3: Additional Helpful Resources in the Practice of EBLM 191

Appendices 227

Appendix A. Appropriate Study Design 229

Appendix B. Classifying Levels of Evidence According to Type of Research Question 238

Appendix C. CASP Critical Appraisal Checklist for Diagnostic Tests 239

Appendix D. CASP Critical Appraisal Checklist for Prognostic Studies 242

Appendix E. CASP Critical Appraisal Checklist for Outcome Studies 246

Appendix F. Example of a Worked Critical Appraisal of Impact on Outcomes 249

Appendix G. Generic Checklist for Applying Evidence (Step A4) 255

Appendix H. Test Yourself 258

Index 261

FOREWORD

Why should you bother reading this foreword? If you do, it will provide some background and orientation to the emerging field of Evidence-Based Laboratory Medicine.

As director of the Centre for Evidence-Based Medicine in Oxford, I have had an ongoing interest in how evidence-based practice has evolved beyond "medicine," into surgery, dermatology, pediatrics, physiotherapy, nursing, and social work—to name only a few. Why this interest in evidence-based practice by so many fields? One driving force is the increased, and increasing, complexity of all branches of medicine. Research provides us with new information and new tools, which we must either reject or master. But these riches require some work in sifting and learning. Part of the puzzle of managing the resulting complex decision making is the ability to appraise, understand, and master the research evidence. Of course, "evidence" is but part of the decision-making process, which also involves practicalities, clinical loads, costs, and many other factors. But with the growth in the range and number of tests, evidence about laboratory tests has become critical to both purchasing decisions and clinical advice.

The demands on a laboratory professional's knowledge will increase. In addition to the growth in the range of tests, the role of the laboratory is changing. Point-of-care testing and self-monitoring by patients are but two examples of this change. Those working in laboratory medicine must be skilled at navigating these changes. This means not being swept away by current fashion, but instead taking a critical view of the research and evaluations of new tests and new roles of old tests. Newer is not necessarily better. So an hour of searching and critical appraisal may save months of work and years of regret in implementing inappropriate tests or test processes. This is where evidence-based laboratory medicine plays a vital role.

For those needing an upgrade in the skills of evidence-based practice as applied to laboratory medicine, this workbook is a great place to start. The authors have been pioneers in the field, having run workshops around the world and edited the first textbook on evidence-based laboratory medicine. The book takes the reader through all the traditional steps of evidence-based medicine, but has made the modifications needed to make the techniques applicable and relevant to laboratory medicine. For instance, this book includes, but goes beyond, the traditional diagnostic role of tests. The authors point out that questions arise from many sources: from a single patient's abnormal test result, from clinicians' general uncertainty about unfamiliar tests, or from policy issues arising from the constant flow of new test methods and processes. They also recognize that there are many other purposes of tests, such as prognosis, screening, and, perhaps most importantly, clinical monitoring. The latter may well be the fastest-growing area of the laboratory workload as we encounter an aging population surviving longer with chronic diseases such as ischemic heart disease, heart failure, and diabetes. Laboratories are well poised to take a major role in this area, by providing better clinical guidance and even acting as the central point of communication for some monitoring problems, such as INR testing. Again, an evidence-based approach will be pivotal to sensible management of this transition.

So I assume if you have read this foreword, you will read the workbook (or indeed may have already read it!). So what then? I would suggest you quickly move to regularly trying the methods. Keep a list of issues and questions that come up each week, and then aim to perform searches and appraisals on some of the most critical ones. If these turn out to be important, you might like to share your findings in a team "journal club." This shouldn't consist of a haphazard scan of *Clinical Chemistry* or the *Annals of Clinical Biochemistry*, but rather a filtering and focus on important clinical or purchasing issues of the laboratory. Evidence-based laboratory medicine is a tool for better decision making, and that needs practice.

So I wish you well with this endeavor, and trust you will find how it benefits your own learning, your clinical colleagues, and—most importantly—the patients that the laboratory is ultimately helping to receive better care.

Professor Paul Glasziou
Director, Centre for Evidence-Based Medicine
University of Oxford
Oxford, UK

PREFACE

"A prudent question is one-half of wisdom." —Sir Francis Bacon

The process of clinicians seeing patients is about "problem resolution" and decision making *(1)*; the decisions may involve screening, diagnosis, prognosis, or treatment—and the decisions should be based on evidence, patient values, and resources *(2)*. Similarly, the process of healthcare policy making is about "problem resolution" and decision making; the decisions should be based on evidence, values, and resources *(2)*. The role of laboratory medicine in the patient's healthcare journey is to assist in "problem resolution" and the use of the service should likewise be based on evidence, values, and resources. Experience will also play a key role in the decision making.

Sackett et al. *(3)* described Evidence-Based Medicine (EBM) as "the conscientious, explicit, and judicious use of current best evidence in making decisions about the care of individual patients." Guyatt et al. *(4, 5)* have stated that an evidence-based approach to the practice of medicine, and laboratory medicine, involves two fundamental facets:

1. that evidence alone is not sufficient, and
2. that there is a hierarchy of evidence that should be used to guide decision making.

The first facet points out that in making a decision, the evidence must be balanced together with benefits and risks, as well as the inconveniences and costs, associated with a specific decision. In other words, clinical judgment is required with respect to how evidence is used in making decisions. Thus, evidence has to be put into the context of the individual patient and the clinical setting. The second facet recognizes that the evidence used to inform decisions must be of adequate quality. In our earlier writings we have taken Sackett's definition and defined Evidence-Based Laboratory Medicine (EBLM) as "the conscientious, explicit, and judicious use of best evidence in the use of laboratory medicine investigations for assisting in making decisions about the care of individual patients" *(5)*.

Edward Hodnett, in his book *The Art of Problem Solving*, observed that

> *If you don't ask the right questions, you don't get the right answers. A question asked in the right way often points to its own answer. Asking questions is the ABC of diagnosis. Only the inquiring mind solves problems* (6).

It follows that if you don't get the right answer, then the decision is likely to be unsatisfactory.

We would add this: that a question is an expression of an unresolved problem.

Laboratorians must remember that clinicians are trained to think in terms of Bayes' theorem, i.e., *Post-test odds = Pre-test odds × likelihood ratio*. Thus, for a test to be clinically useful, the prevalence of disease in the target population must be known, as this is directly related to pre-test odds. Further, the result of the test must be related to the likelihood of disease. This therefore provides us with a definition for that elusive concept of the "appropriate test"—one in which the result has a good chance of providing an answer to the question, or perhaps more accurately stated, increases the odds that an answer to the problem is correct. Pursuing this argument raises a number of issues, including that the clinician knows four things:

1. the question to ask,
2. the decision to be made with the result produced—whether the result be normal or abnormal,
3. the action that should be taken when the decision has been made, and
4. the expected outcome—which might include benefit and risk to the patient, and cost to the healthcare provider.

The laboratorian, when responding to the clinician's need (test request), also needs to know the question that is being asked. In the past it was suggested that the clinician write the question—rather than the tests—on the request (or order) form, so that the most appropriate tests are requested. In fact this does happen sometimes, e.g., the request is simply "myeloma?" The laboratorian providing the service to the clinician will also have questions in relation to the appropriateness of the services provided, including whether it

1. meets the clinician's needs,
2. is of the necessary quality and cost, and
3. benefits the patient.

The healthcare service provider, the purchaser (commissioner), and the policymaker will also have questions in relation to the services that are provided—Are they effective? Are they efficient? Sir Francis Bacon's observation remains very apt!

The application of EBLM to daily practice comprises five steps, referred to as the EBLM A5 Cycle:

1. Ask
2. Acquire
3. Appraise
4. Apply
5. Assess (or Audit) *(7)*.

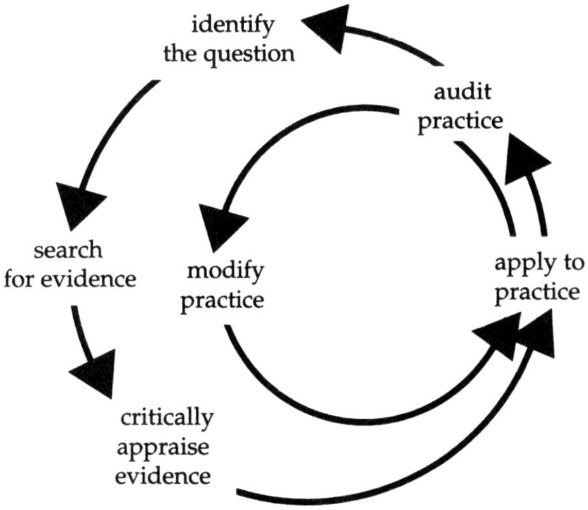

Reprinted with permission from Price CP. Evidence-based laboratory medicine: supporting decision-making. Clin Chem 2000;46:1041–50.

In that the question will often lead to new knowledge, this is a process of continuous learning. The purpose of this book is to take the reader step-by-step through the process of finding and using evidence (knowledge) to solve the problems that arise on a day-to-day basis in the practice of laboratory medicine. It is intended as a learning tool for the laboratorian, not just when embarking on a career in laboratory medicine, but for continuous learning. The reader is encouraged to add his/her own experiences as part of a continuous learning process; this will then provide a valuable resource to share with others, e.g., trainees, in the future as part of mentoring.

One of the reasons for writing this book was provided by feedback during an EBLM workshop. One attendee observed that the course had provided the structure to clinical biochemistry that his earlier training had lacked—it put the science into context. Another delegate, however, admitted she did not know where she would apply all the skills she had just learned. (In many ways this is a very reasonable observation when you start to think about all of the problems or challenges that can arise in one's daily laboratory practice; all those questions to answer!) We also realized that our earlier book was more of a textbook and that what was needed was a more practical workbook.

We were aware of Sharon Straus' *(8)* and Paul Glasziou's *(9)* books on how to practice EBM, and we felt that a similar approach was needed for laboratory medicine. We talked to Paul about our idea and he encouraged us to go ahead. We would like to recognize the valuable advice that Paul has given us in the preparation of this book, with many helpful comments on early drafts. We have enjoyed taking our experiences through the EBLM A5 Cycle, and in so doing it has opened our eyes to the complexity of our specialty, the need to better understand the clinician's needs, and to learn how to work better with purchasers (commissioners) and policymakers.

There are obvious challenges to writing this kind of "virtual" instruction, and it has been our great pleasure that Joanne Lozar Glenn agreed to join us in this venture. Joanne has a Master's degree in Education, and is an educational and editorial consultant. She is an instructor by training and practice, and thrives on developing, designing, and delivering courses and other educational products and services. Her input has been crucial in converting our approach to writing into a more interactive style.

We would also like to thank Joanna Grimes of AACC Press for her expert guidance and unfailing commitment to the production of this book. It has been a real pleasure to work with her.

We hope that you, the reader, find this guide helpful in bringing EBLM into your daily practice, and that it helps with the challenges that you face.

Christopher P. Price
Robert H. Christenson
November 2008

References

1. Del Mar C, Doust J, Glasziou P. Clinical Thinking: Evidence, Communication and Decision-Making. Oxford: Blackwell Publishing BMJ Books, 2006:127pp.

2. Muir Gray JA. Evidence-Based Healthcare: How to Make Health Policy and Management Decisions, 2nd ed. Edinburgh: Churchill Livingstone, 2001:444pp.

3. Sackett DL, Rosenberg WM, Gray JA, et al. Evidence-based medicine: what it is and what it isn't. BMJ 1996;312:71–2.

4. Guyatt G, Haynes B, Jaeschke R, et al. Introduction: the philosophy of evidence-based medicine. In: Guyatt G, Rennie D, eds. User's Guide to the Medical Literature: A Manual for Evidence-Based Clinical Practice. Chicago: JAMA and Archive Journals, American Medical Association, 2002:3–12.

5. Price CP, Christenson RH, eds. Evidence-Based Laboratory Medicine, 2nd ed. Washington, DC: AACC Press, 2007:545pp.

6. Hodnett E. The Art of Problem Solving: How to Improve Your Methods. New York, NY: Harper, 1955:202pp.

7. Price CP. Evidence-based laboratory medicine: supporting decision-making. Clin Chem 2000;46:1041–50.

8. Straus S, Richardson WS, Glasziou P, Haynes RB. Evidence-Based Medicine: How to Practice and Teach EBM, 3rd ed. Edinburgh: Elsevier Churchill Livingstone, 2005:299pp.

9. Glasziou P, Del Mar C, Salisbury J. Evidence-Based Practice Workbook, 2nd ed. Oxford: Blackwell Publishing BMJ Books, 2007:202pp.

About This Book: What to Expect and How to Use It

You have probably become very familiar with the phrases "Evidence-Based Medicine or EBM," "Evidence-Based Laboratory Medicine or EBLM," and "Evidence-Based Practice or EBP." Still, you may be wondering how these terms apply to you in your day-by-day professional practice. This book can help.

Here's What to Expect

You are about to learn how to apply the principles of EBLM. Applying these principles has several benefits:

You will become a more effective member of the healthcare team. Our own experience with EBLM has given us a structure that helps us fulfill our roles as members of the clinical team caring for patients, leaders of a key service provider to that team, and members of the healthcare provider's management team.

You will become a more effective problem solver. One of our key roles as laboratorians is to help solve problems. Applying EBLM has helped us become better practitioners, clinical researchers, and educators as we've learned to more precisely identify the problem, find or develop the evidence, and communicate the answer to the inquirer. The Institute of Medicine, in its study of the U.S. healthcare system, concluded that poor communication was one of the major causes of medical errors. Working through this guide will improve your ability to deal with the problems you face in your daily professional practice.

Your work will contribute more effectively to improving healthcare outcomes. The core principles of EBM and EBLM are the same, as are the core objectives. Both disciplines emphasize improving the quality of information to support decision making—moving attention *away from understanding the mechanisms of disease and toward improving outcomes.*

In laboratory medicine this is a significant paradigm shift. It also represents a major paradigm shift at managerial and policymaking levels, because of its emphasis on how the laboratory can benefit the patient, the clinician or caregiver, and the provider organization. Because these are major paradigm shifts, they are also major challenges, but we believe they represent an acknowledgment that cost and quality are both major issues in healthcare today—and so value becomes paramount.

What You'll Learn

There are five steps to EBLM—**the EBLM A5 Cycle**—and they represent a logical sequence that begins with a statement of the healthcare problem. Here are the five steps, and what you'll learn to do in each one:

1. **ASK:** How to structure the question that states the problem in a way that enables you to move on to the next step.
2. **ACQUIRE:** How to find the evidence that might answer the question.
3. **APPRAISE:** How to determine whether the evidence is reliable, and if it can be used to answer the question.
4. **APPLY:** How to take the evidence and apply it to your problem.
5. **ASSESS or AUDIT:** How to assess the process you have used and determine its effectiveness.

How You'll Learn

We want this to be a practical, useful workbook. So we're going to introduce you to the application of EBLM in a number of different scenarios—from answering a telephone inquiry to establishing policy for the use of a particular test.

You'll explore case studies that illustrate the principles of EBLM in diverse applications. You'll observe situations in your own institution and consider how they might be addressed using the principles of EBLM. You'll formulate research questions and then follow those questions to their evidence-based solutions.

As much as possible, given the confines and limitations of a printed text, you'll be involved in "action learning" and be provided with additional resources you can investigate for further information.

What You'll Be Able to Do As a Result

- **Learn how to structure questions to help with problem solving**
- **Search the literature effectively and efficiently**
- **Critically appraise evidence effectively and efficiently**

- **Answer questions** concerning
  - background to a condition or test (etiology)
  - preanalytical considerations for tests
  - interpretation of results
  - action to take upon receipt of results
- **Prepare guidance for clinicians** on the use of tests
  - for screening
  - for diagnosis
  - for prognosis
  - for treatment selection
  - for treatment optimization
  - for treatment compliance
- **Prepare a case for a new test,** and state
  - the impact of test use on clinical outcome
  - the modality of testing and impact on outcomes
  - how practice should change
  - the economic benefit of using the test
- **Make healthcare policy,** including taking into account
  - the health economics of testing
- **Perform research** and create
  - a study design to investigate any of the above items
- **Communicate with your colleagues more effectively**
  - in the laboratory,
  - on wards or in clinics, and
  - in the boardroom . . .

. . . because you will have a better understanding of the problems and know how to obtain the solutions.

You'll also be able to do all of this more quickly and efficiently. This can be a great asset when answering the telephone, where you may not know what problem is going to be thrown at you.

How This Book Is Organized

The book is divided into three parts:

- **Introduction and context-setting.**
- **The step-by-step guide** to the EBLM A5 cycle.
- **Supporting information,** including a glossary of key terms, useful calculations, a list of websites, and sources of evidence and guidelines for incorporating EBLM into your practice.

Each part contains a "roadmap" to what the section will cover. Content is organized into main points and supporting details that help you understand the material and processes you'll be asked to apply. In addition, we've included sidebars that provide supplementary information about the material covered, and key concepts you'll want to understand.

Case studies are the core resource of the book and when they appear, you are encouraged to work through the examples (cases), follow the reasoning used to address the problem and find a solution, and then add your own cases for analysis and evaluation. Finally, you'll be given regular opportunities to pause, reflect, and assess what you've learned.

How to Use This Book

We have organized this book so that

- You will see how EBLM has been applied in a range of scenarios.
- You can see how each step of the process is accomplished.
- You get the chance to perform each step yourself on new cases.
- You can create your own cases from your own experiences.
- You can add additional resources (for example, from the medical literature).
- You can evaluate your own experience with applying the principles of EBLM (this is crucial) as well as the effectiveness of its application in your workplace.

Certainly you can work through each of the examples in your own time and in your own way.

Yet we believe this book should not only be a resource for your own education and training, but also for that of your colleagues. The EBLM cases that you develop can be shared with others (sharing best practice) and also can help you in a mentoring role with new members of staff. You could even develop your own EBLM training course, based on your own case studies.

If you get stuck and don't think you have the answer, then be bold! Take your problem to a colleague and discuss it—you may both learn from the experience. You could even use this approach as the framework for regular case conferences in your department—to structure all of your discussions, or to facilitate a problem-solving meeting.

Part 1

An Introduction to Evidence-Based Laboratory Medicine (EBLM)

In this chapter

- EBLM in the clinical laboratory: six key challenges
- Key elements of clinical decision making
- Relevance of evidence: formulating a properly structured question
- The need for EBLM
- The A5 cycle for practicing EBLM
- The skills needed to practice EBLM
- Uses of EBLM in daily practice
- Coming full circle: key learning points

EBLM in the Clinical Laboratory: Six Key Challenges

The director of the hospital's intensive care unit (ICU) is implementing tight glycemic control for patients on the unit. He asks the ICU's clinical chemistry liaison which glucose measurement system he should be using.

The choice lies between providing a rapid central laboratory service or using point-of-care testing (POCT). The options for POCT amount to either the use of a hand-held patient glucose system or using the glucose module on the benchtop blood gas and electrolyte analyzer.

What do you advise, and why?

❖❖❖

Your laboratory receives a request from the local nephrologist to start measuring cystatin C, because it appears to provide a better estimate of glomerular filtration rate than serum creatinine. If you were the laboratory director, what would you do?

❖❖❖

A cardiologist visits the laboratory to inquire about providing B-type natriuretic peptide tests in the clinic to help him guide his management of newly diagnosed patients with heart failure. If you were the laboratory director, what would you tell him?

❖❖❖

A public health physician from a local health maintenance organization (HMO) writes to the head of the laboratory, indicating that he wants to explore the potential benefits of using POCT for HbA1c in the diabetes center clinics. The physician has heard that improved outcomes can be achieved using this approach, and that this approach helps involve patients in the management of their condition. He asks if there is any evidence on the use of POCT for HbA1c. He also broaches the possibility of moving some diabetes care into the primary care setting. The head of the laboratory asks you to deal with the issue. What would you do?

❖❖❖

The chief executive of your hospital is concerned that the recorded times for length of stay for patients attending the emergency department are increasing, especially at peak times. He calls a meeting of the emergency department staff and the directors of the laboratory and imaging departments. Their charge: to find ways of improving triage times throughout the department. If you were the laboratory director, how would you proceed?

❖❖❖

A local HMO policymaker is investigating the possibility of implementing a screening program for Chlamydia *infection following reports of an increase in the complication rates associated with the infection. An initial conversation with the local microbiologist raises the question as to the best screening method to use, with the recommendation that a DNA amplification method would be the best choice. What would you suggest?*

❖❖❖

These situations call for a process of decision making that goes beyond mere "experience." This process is called evidence-based laboratory medicine (EBLM), which has its roots in evidence-based medicine (EBM).

Each of these situations above reflects different challenges or problems—namely analytical performance, diagnostic accuracy, monitoring and outcomes, operational change and outcomes,

What Is Evidence-Based Medicine (EBM)? Key Definitions and Observations

EBM involves

- the conscientious, explicit and judicious use of current best evidence in making decisions about the care of individual patients *(1)*
- the integration of best research evidence with clinical expertise and patient values *(2)*
- trying to improve the quality of the information on which decisions are based *(3)*
- thinking not about mechanisms but about outcomes *(3)*

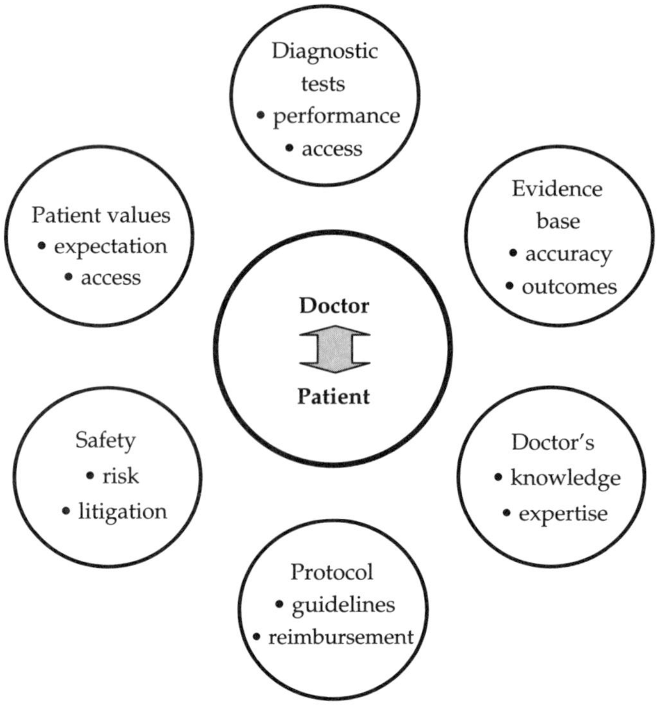

Key elements of decision making and the use of laboratory investigations

operational change and health economics, and policymaking, respectively. In each situation, laboratorians used principles of EBLM to answer questions and solve problems that arose in the use of the laboratory medicine service. They searched for the best evidence, based on scientific studies, about how each diagnostic method impacted the health outcomes of individual patients.

In this workbook, you'll learn how to apply these principles to your work in the laboratory, so that diagnostic tests are used appropriately to make better healthcare decisions.

Key Concept

EBM and EBLM are about translating evidence into practice.

Key Elements of Clinical Decision Making

We can think of EBM as a culture that underpins the daily practice of medicine and embraces a range of concepts and philosophies. Let's look at each of these concepts in detail.

Evidence: the information that gives grounds for belief; that which points to, reveals or suggests something. ***Best evidence*** reflects the quality of the information on which we base decisions. We focus on clinical decisions we need to make today, which means using the best, most up-to-date *available* evidence, not waiting for the best *possible* evidence.

The quality, and value, of information: which depends on the quality of the "raw" evidence, its reporting, its interpretation, and its relevance. Obtaining high quality, valuable information means minimizing bias in the generation, reporting, and interpretation of experimental results, as well as in the way that the results are incorporated into information databases (e.g., clinical guidelines and care pathways). Some of these issues will be highlighted in later sections, e.g., in critical appraisal of evidence. (See also Part 3, "Bias" and "Validity.")

Integration of evidence with clinical expertise: Information is the basis for managing patient care. But information must be integrated with clinical expertise—the combination of clinical skills and experience supported by knowledge and an understanding of how to apply it. Evolving expertise assumes a transition from a dependence on background knowledge (the basic science of a disease) to an application of foreground knowledge (see sidebar, "Background and Foreground Information," page 7)—the experience gained from applying best evidence to the care of individual patients, which brings to the forefront their variable characteristics, the variability in disease presentation and evolution and in how patients respond to therapies, as well as their individual values and choices *(4)*.

Patient values: The Evidence-Based Medicine Working Group has described values and preferences as "the underlying processes we bring to bear in weighing what our patients and our society will gain—or lose—when we make a management decision" *(2)*.

Bias and Chance

It is important to understand the difference between bias and chance. Bias is the result of a systematic error, whereas chance leads to a random error or variation. Chance, however, is not systematic and so is harder to describe and recognize; the analytical equivalent is imprecision.

The "fundamental equation of error" is

observed results = true result + bias + noise

Noise in a study can be reduced by increasing the sample numbers, whereas in the case of bias a good study design is needed (Paul Glasziou personal communication).

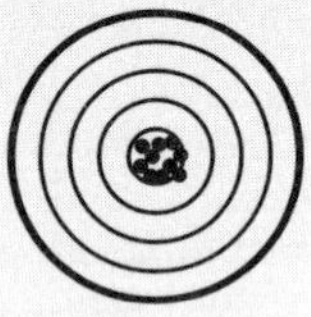

accurate and precise

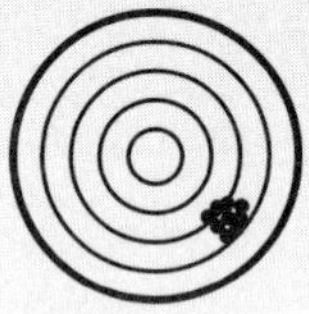

inaccurate but precise

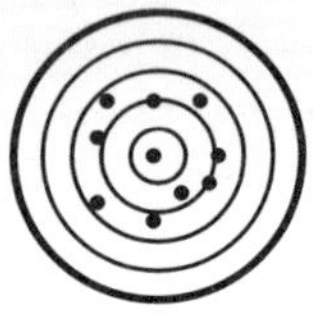

accurate but imprecise

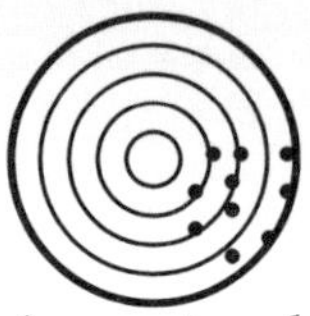

inaccurate and imprecise

Value judgments about clinical treatment happen in a broad landscape: from whether the test or treatment interventions are worth the cost; to whether the tests and therapies are effective, given that evidence of effectiveness is predominantly gathered from a large cohort of similar, yet different, patients; to what the patient prefers regarding involvement in decision making. (Some examples: participation in a Down syndrome screening program, the management of type 1 diabetes in children and adolescents, POCT for HbA1c when patients have been unwilling to perform self-monitoring of blood glucose.)

Outcomes not mechanisms: Physicians have been trained in "background information," i.e., the basic science of a disease. However, the physician managing an individual patient needs "foreground information," i.e., the experience gained from applying best evidence to the care of individual patients. Laboratorians use this kind of information to make better decisions about testing, so they can help clinicians make a correct diagnosis and initiate appropriate treatment, the goal being an improved outcome.

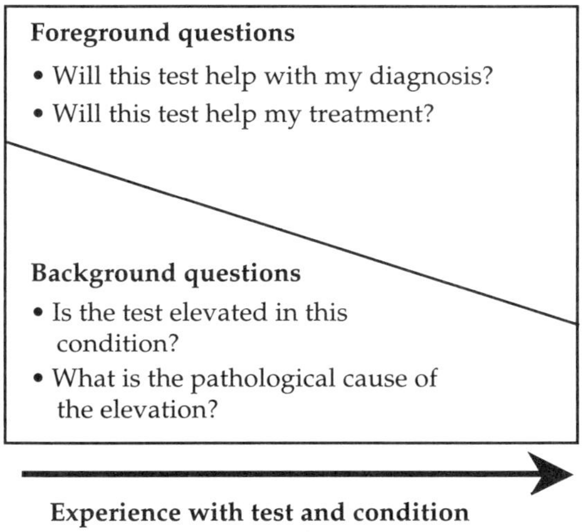

Background and foreground information: questions from basic science to improving outcomes

Key Concept

Clinical decision making focuses on the *conscientious, explicit,* and *judicious use* of best evidence. By recognizing diligence and thoroughness, clarity in statement, and prudence of purpose, this use of evidence provides a quality framework for the underlying principles of EBM—from understanding the clinical problem, or question, right through to applying the evidence.

Background and Foreground Information

Different medical professionals need different types of evidence, or information, to contribute meaningfully in their field. If you are a basic research scientist in the field of drug discovery, then you will want to know all about the underlying pathobiology of a specific disease, and the biochemical aberrations at the organ, cellular, and molecular levels. If you work in biomarker development, you will want to understand the nature of the marker, i.e., its structure, and its relationship to the disease of interest. This evidence provides what has been called "*background information*" or the "*basic science*" of the disease. However it does not give you much information about how to manage the patient sitting in front of the physician in his consulting room, or lying on a bed in the emergency department.

The evidence that helps resolve these types of problems is called "*foreground information*" and is designed to meet a clinical need, to help the clinician deal effectively, efficiently, and compassionately with individual patients.

More junior health professionals are likely to depend more on background information at the outset of their careers, and as they gain experience then they will move forward to using experience and more foreground information. This is, in part, because the teaching of clinical medicine has always emphasized the underpinning science; this is beginning to change as the principles of EBM are taught early in the medical school curriculum.

Relevant Evidence in Clinical Decision Making: The Importance of Formulating a Properly Structured Question

Relevance of evidence seems to be so obvious that stating it may make you feel insulted. Yet we know from systematic literature reviews that many papers are rejected from further consideration because the evidence is not relevant to the situation in hand. There are many simple examples: applying data gathered on patients in secondary care to patients in primary care, applying data gathered in one ethnic group to another, etc.

One way to ensure relevance in the clinical setting is to provide a properly structured question when investigating a clinical problem. Richardson et al. *(5)* proposed a simple system for reformulating general questions, which required four key pieces of information—relevant identification of

1. the (**P**)atient or (**P**)opulation,
2. the (**I**)ntervention,
3. the (**C**)ontrol, and
4. the (**O**)utcome.

The acronym **PICO** is now commonly used and is the subject of the first section of Part 2 of this book, which outlines the steps in applying EBLM. There are also some derivatives of the PICO approach and you will be introduced to these in Part 2.

Key Concepts

A question is an expression of an unresolved problem. A request for a laboratory test should always be looked on as helping a clinician to deal with an unresolved problem–and the result helping to provide an answer.

Test results are only useful if they are "reviewed and used" to help make decisions about patient care. Some literature shows that many results are not reviewed, and even more not used to help make patient care decisions.

Evidence-Based Healthcare

EBM is not just for clinical decision making. Its underlying principles are also increasingly employed in healthcare management and policymaking.

Pressures in the form of increasing patient expectations, an aging population, the availability of new technologies, and the disparities in healthcare provision around the world have meant that most governments are looking at ways to make better use of available resources to meet these needs. There is also a widespread recognition that medical interventions have associated risks, and that errors occur in healthcare delivery. Consequently the core objectives of EBM are maximizing benefit and minimizing risks, at reasonable cost—and about "doing the right thing, right" *(6)*.

It is always helpful, therefore, to be aware that the skills learned in relation to the practice of EBM apply at the level of the individual patient's care, right through to service leadership and management. These principles are therefore applicable to the practice of laboratory medicine.

Pause and Reflect

Given this introduction to EBM in clinical decision making, brainstorm some of the parallels you see between EBM and applying EBM principles in laboratory medicine (EBLM).

....

....

....

....

....

....

....

....

....

....

....

....

What Is Evidence-Based Laboratory Medicine (EBLM)?

The definitions applied to EBM can equally be applied to EBLM with a slight modification to the original definition of Sackett et al. *(1, 7)*:

- "the conscientious, explicit, and judicious use of **current best evidence** on **diagnostic tests** in **making decisions** about the **care of individual patients**."

All of the other statements about EBM made earlier apply equally to EBLM. Again, let's look at these items in more detail.

Best evidence: Sackett and Haines *(8)* clearly described an architecture for diagnostic research studies. This architecture demonstrated the links between background and foreground information and the quality of the information gleaned from different types of studies in relation to the needs of healthcare professionals. Four levels of research studies (in the form of questions) were described:

1. **Demonstrating the relationship between the test and the disease,** i.e., "Do patients with the target disorder have different results from normal individuals?"
2. **Assessing the likelihood of association between the test result and the disease,** i.e., "Are patients with certain test results more likely to have the target disorder than patients with other test results?"
3. **Assessing whether the test could distinguish those patients at risk of developing the disease,** i.e., "Among patients in whom it is clinically sensible to suspect the target disorder, does the level of the test result distinguish those with and without the target disorder?"
4. **Assessing whether those patients who had access to the test achieved a better health outcome,** i.e., "Do patients who undergo this diagnostic test fare better (in their ultimate health outcomes) than similar patients who do not?"

The appropriate diagnostic test: There is a great deal of concern about appropriate testing. Most of the literature focuses on "over-use," with only limited attention given to "under-use." Invariably, appropriate use is also linked with demand management, and again the emphasis is on minimizing unnecessary testing, for which there are a number of approaches *(7)*.

Background

Relation between pathology and identification of marker

Measurement of marker: analytical and biological variation

Relation to disease activity: results in affected patients differ from normals

Patients with certain results are more likely to have the condition

Results differentiate those with the condition from those without the condition

Patients having the test have better outcomes than those not having the test

Foreground

The hierarchy of evidence from characterizing method performance to demonstrating benefit to the patient

However an "appropriate test" can be defined as "the provision of a diagnostic test result in response to a clinical question, that should enable a decision to be made, leading to an action being taken, and which will yield an improved health outcome" *(7)*. You will see that appropriateness is judged in a very different way. The improved health outcome, as discussed below, may be for the patient, the healthcare professional, the healthcare provider, or the healthcare purchaser.

Decision making: Much of the evidence base in laboratory medicine contributes more to background information than foreground information. For example, it describes the analytical performance of a test and the correlation between marker levels and the existence and severity of disease *(8)*, as well as providing information on the diagnostic accuracy of a test. It provides less information on how use of the test helps to make better decisions. Clearly, making a healthcare decision is based on there being a problem or a question that is being asked in the first place. This can be viewed as a series of issues to be resolved (questions) against which you can quickly judge the validity—or appropriateness—of any test request order:

- What is the problem?
- What is the question being asked?
- What decision are you likely to make?
- What action will you take?
- What is the expected outcome?

Satisfactory answers to all of these questions could be considered to constitute the criteria for an appropriate test. It is implied that the additional investment is worthwhile.

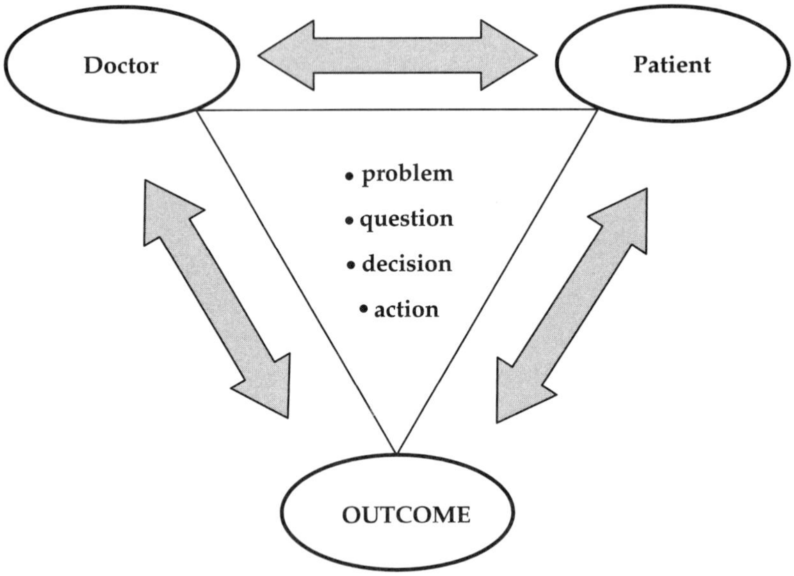

Patient-centered decision making: from problem to outcome

Impact on care of individual patients (outcomes): Sackett and Haines *(8)* highlighted the importance of recognizing that the best evidence of test effectiveness was that which showed ***whether patients who had access to a test fared better in terms of outcomes than those who did not have access to the test***. Clearly "access" in this context includes correct interpretation of the result, with the right decision being made and the right action taken.

Fryback and Thornbury *(9)* stated that "patient outcome data are the *sine qua non* of efficacy from the individual patient's perspective." They also described a hierarchy of evidence that ranged from technical performance to impact on outcomes, encompassing all the evidence

Applying "PICO" to a Real-Life Scenario

Recall the introductory scenario (pp. 3–4) in which recorded times for length of stay in the emergency department are increasing. The hospital's chief executive asked for ways to improve triage times. One hypothesis was that rapid delivery of results, using POCT, would provide a solution.

Asking the five "generic" questions necessary for decision making helps define the question in "PICO" terms. Thus,

1. **The problem** is increased length of stay in the emergency department.
2. **The question** is will POCT help solve the problem.
3. **The decision you are likely to make** is that if using POCT will produce a benefit, then introduce POCT.
4. **The action you will take**, given a positive answer to the question (#2), is to introduce POCT.
5. **The expected outcome** is a reduction in the length of stay in the emergency department.

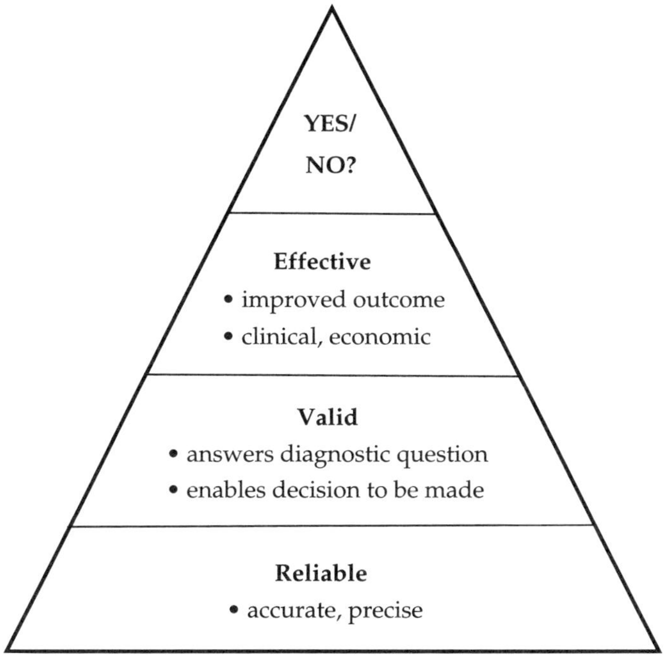

The hierarchy of evidence from assessing method performance to introduction

required to decide to invest in the test, i.e., the presentation of a business case.

This "business case" approach differentiates between clinical, operational, and economic outcomes:

- *Clinical outcomes* focus primarily on the patient but will be of interest to clinicians, caregivers, and other healthcare professionals as well as to service purchasers and providers. The primary measures of clinical outcome are mortality and morbidity (the 5Ds—death, disease, disability, discomfort, and dissatisfaction!). A range of surrogate measures can be used to assess clinical outcomes, many of which are used routinely in clinical practice, e.g., HbA1c as a measure of glycemic control, and urine albumin creatinine ratio as an early indicator of diabetic nephropathy.
- *Operational outcomes* are often considered a part of economic outcomes. We have separated them to highlight operational changes that must be effected and measured to ensure that benefits are achieved. This can be particularly helpful when planning the introduction of a new test, or a new approach to testing, e.g., POCT. Operational outcomes can be measured in terms of resource utilization as well as in the efficiency of the patient or care pathway. Examples include changes in staff requirement, equipment, and space utilization, e.g., from a

reduction in clinic visits and in length of stay, to conversion to day-case surgery (at the provider level) and reduction in time taken off work to attend clinics (at the patient level).

- *Economic outcomes* are focused on the resources required to provide care, which again can be examined at the service provider level as well as at the purchaser and societal levels. At the service provider level, service resource allocation is often undertaken in "silos," e.g., for laboratory medicine or imaging services, which constitutes the most narrow, or "lowest" perspective. It is more effective to look at broader, or "higher," perspectives, namely the impact on either the recipient of test results, e.g., the emergency department, or levels such as the hospital and/or local health economy. Deeks *(10)* delineated surrogate outcome measures into "clinical" and "process," and some examples of surrogate outcome measures are given in the table below.

Surrogate Measures of Clinical and Process Outcome

Clinical outcome measure	Application	Process outcome measure	Application
Complication rate	Effectiveness of glycemic control in intensive care	Length of stay	Effectiveness of POCT, e.g., cardiac markers, in the emergency department
Readmission rate	Intra-operative parathyroid hormone measurement	Number of clinic visits	Effectiveness of POCT for HbA1c in managing diabetes
HbA1c	Effectiveness of glycemic control	Caregiver's time	Use of POCT for rapid decision making, e.g., in the emergency department
Bone marker	Effectiveness of anti-resorptive agents	Transfer of care from secondary to primary care sector	Effectiveness of POCT in managing diabetes
Urine albumin: creatinine ratio	Early indicator of diabetic nephropathy	Choice of diagnostic modality	Use of B-type natriuretic peptide to rule out need for echocardiography in all dyspneic patients
Cholesterol	Effectiveness of statin therapy	Reduce need for laboratory tests	Urinalysis by strip test to rule out UTI
B-type natriuretic peptide	Effectiveness of treatment for heart failure		

EBLM Fosters Good Practice, Quality Specifications, and Decision Making

Good practice in laboratory medicine necessarily operates at four levels:

1. **Analytically,** i.e., that the test meets the prescribed quality specifications (background questions and information).
2. **Clinically,** i.e., that the right test was ordered, the right interpretation made, the right decision made, and the right action taken.
3. **Operationally,** which can be considered as five interrelated levels: (i) at the patient level, the correct specimen is taken at the right time; (ii) at the laboratory level, the specimen is transported, handled, analyzed, and reported correctly; (iii) at the clinician level, the sequence of events from request to action is seamless; (iv) at the organizational level all the activities operate in a complementary (i.e., "connected") fashion; and finally, (v) if a new test or procedure is introduced, that the necessary changes to the care pathway are made.
4. **Economically,** which can be considered in terms of the costs of providing the test and the savings that can be made through the use of the test.

The validation of analytical performance and its application in routine practice are recognized through quality systems such as the Clinical Laboratory Improvement Act (CLIA) *(11)*. Only then is it possible to move to foreground questions related to decision making and outcomes.

However, compared with clinical EBM—e.g., in the case of therapies—less evidence links the performance of diagnostic tests with decision making. In part this is because the types of studies performed on diagnostic tests usually rely on analysis of retrospective (stored) samples—which by definition means that the results have not been used as part of the clinical decision-making process, and thus the role in improving health outcomes cannot be assessed.

It is pointless and inappropriate to perform a test if it does not provide an answer to a clinical question (addressing a clinical need) that can then inform decision making *(7, 12)*. This notwithstanding, the clinical performance of tests for decision making is firmly based on the information provided by background studies.

Key Concept

The best evidence on the effectiveness of a test is that which shows whether patients who had access to a test fared better (in terms of outcomes) than those who did not have access to the test.

Pause and Reflect

Thinking about your own laboratory experience, rate the emphasis/attention paid to applying EBLM-related principles in daily practice (0 = none; 5 = moderate; 10 = full):

Commitment to best available evidence 0 10

Relentless focus on appropriate testing 0 10

Use of foreground vs. background information in clinical decision making 0 10

Outcomes vs. testing mechanisms 0 10

Are there ways to "move the bar" in the direction of applying EBLM principles? ....

....

....

....

....

....

....

....

....

....

....

....

....

Why Do We Need EBLM?

As Sharon Strauss and colleagues so ably point out in their book *Evidence-Based Medicine: How to Practice and Teach EBM (13),* the up-to-date, valid information needed to make effective clinical treatment decisions is often inadequate, unavailable, or too cumbersome to achieve. They describe the evolution of EBM in terms of "four realizations" (see sidebar, "The Evolution of EBM"). They argued that five developments have helped to improve this situation: (i) strategies for searching and appraising evidence, (ii) systematic reviews, (iii) evidence-based summary services, (iv) efficient information systems, and (v) development of a culture of life-long learning (see sidebar on page 18).

This is also true about the information needed in the clinical laboratory regarding what laboratorians need to know about tests before recommending their use. We should be considering specific issues to ensure that we make the best use of laboratory services:

- Clinicians and other health professionals regularly use laboratory investigations in managing their patients and yet **tests are often used inappropriately**.
- **"Inappropriateness" occurs** at the test-requesting phase (**pre-analytically**) and also at the decision-making and application phases (**post-analytically**). Sometimes, results are not even accessed or acted upon despite being reported by the laboratory. Whose responsibility is it to deal with this kind of post-analytical problem?
- Most laboratories provide **laboratory handbooks** to help clinicians use the laboratory, but these documents **are invariably difficult to access**—they are paper rather than electronic, and they are often kept at the nurses' station rather than at the bedside or consulting room.
- The handbooks usually present **information by test and samples needed rather than by clinical need or appropriate testing frequency**. This is beginning to change with the improvement in laboratory information systems—although access by clinicians, through order-communication systems, is not universal.
- Laboratory handbooks **rarely include comprehensive information on the interpretation of results**—or a reference back to the primary, or secondary, literature.

The Evolution of EBM (Part 1): Four Realizations

1. There is **a daily need for valid information** about diagnosis, prognosis, therapy, and prevention.
2. **Traditional sources of this information are inadequate** because they are out of date (textbooks), frequently wrong (experts), ineffective (didactic continuing medical education), or too overwhelming in their volume and too variable in their validity for practical use (medical journals).
3. There is a **disparity between diagnostic skills and clinical judgment**, which increase with experience, **and our up-to-date knowledge and clinical performance**, which decline.
4. **We can't afford more than a few seconds per patient** for finding and assimilating this evidence, nor can we/do we set aside more than half an hour per week for general reading and study.

- **Basic clinical laboratory information** (background information) such as reference ranges and assay accuracy **varies**. Consequently if **clinicians** are caring for patients and move between providers, they **risk misinterpreting results**—and so tests have to be repeated.
- The impact of **analytical and patient (biological) variation** on clinical decision making—and hence, health outcomes—**is poorly understood**. Also, there is **little literature on the impact of inaccuracy and imprecision on outcomes**, although reference to the classical description of these parameters clearly shows it is an important issue. Furthermore access to the information on this variability, especially of biological variation, is poor.
- **A large proportion of the evidence base for laboratory medicine describes background information**, either the technology and its performance, e.g., development and evaluation of methods, or the relationship between the marker (test) and the disease, e.g., pathophysiological mechanisms or marker level and disease severity.
- **We need more foreground information**, i.e., the impact of laboratory medicine investigations on health outcomes; the literature in this area is limited. There is also **limited understanding and recognition of the clinical questions** that are being asked when a test is ordered—and the wide range of questions that may be asked. Consequently it then follows that the decisions and actions associated with the answers given to these questions may not always be clear.
- The **methodology for investigating the utility of tests is not as well-focused or mature** as that used in the evaluation of therapeutic interventions.
- The **regulation of laboratory investigations is primarily based on analytical performance and avoidance of harm**, with little emphasis of the impact on health outcomes.
- There are **few incentives for undertaking the foreground (outcome) studies** to demonstrate the benefits of using new laboratory investigations, and consequently **translation into routine practice is very slow**.

The Evolution of EBM (Part 2): Four Realizations

Fortunately, five developments have enabled this poor state of affairs to be improved:

1. The development of **strategies for efficiently tracking down and appraising evidence** (for its validity and relevance).
2. The **creation of systematic reviews** of the effects of healthcare (epitomized by the Cochrane Collaboration) *(14)*.
3. The **creation of evidence-based journals** of secondary publication (which publish the two percent of clinical articles that are both valid and of immediate clinical use) and of evidence-based summary services such as *Clinical Evidence (15)*.
4. The **creation of information systems** for searching these journals and summary services.
5. The **identification and application of effective strategies for lifelong learning** and for improving our clinical performance.

- The optimal situation is invariably to link a test result with a therapeutic intervention or direct management in order to produce an improved outcome. However, **it is complicated to demonstrate the specific contribution of a laboratory investigation** in a robust experimental study.
- Introducing **a new test, or a way of delivering that test, e.g., POCT, generally involves a change in clinical practice** in order to deliver the benefit, e.g., introduction of a *Chlamydia* screening program to reduce the incidence of complications associated with the infection.

Five key areas arise from this critical analysis, i.e., the need to

1. **Ensure understanding of why tests are used in the management of patients.** This should include the range of clinical questions that are being asked—i.e., that they reflect the clinical needs.
2. **Understand the decisions and the actions** that follow from the answers provided.
3. **Generate evidence** that shows whether these needs can be met (questions answered), and demonstrate the utility of the test and the impact on health outcomes.
4. **Disseminate the evidence** to clinicians, caregivers, and other healthcare professionals in a succinct way that complements their workflow. Consider providing electronic laboratory handbooks with search capabilities based on clinical problems, decision support systems, systematic reviews, clinical guidelines, and care pathways—as well as incorporating the laboratorian as a full member of the clinical team.
5. **Translate high-quality evidence of effectiveness into an objective assessment of health outcomes.** This information can be used in business cases and implementation strategies to enable more effective translation into practice.

Applied EBLM promises to meet these needs and lead to improved clinical outcomes for patients—which is, after all, the point. For EBLM to be effective, the laboratorian must become competent in a number of skills—and know when to use them. These skills comprise the "A5 Cycle."

What You Need to Know about Tests before Recommending Their Use

- Disease mechanism and maker
- Analytical variation
- Biological variation
- Relation between marker and disease activity
- Likelihood of having disease with result X
- What separates those with disease from those without disease?
- Does providing the test give better outcomes?

Also refer again to figure on page 11.

The A5 Cycle for Practicing EBLM

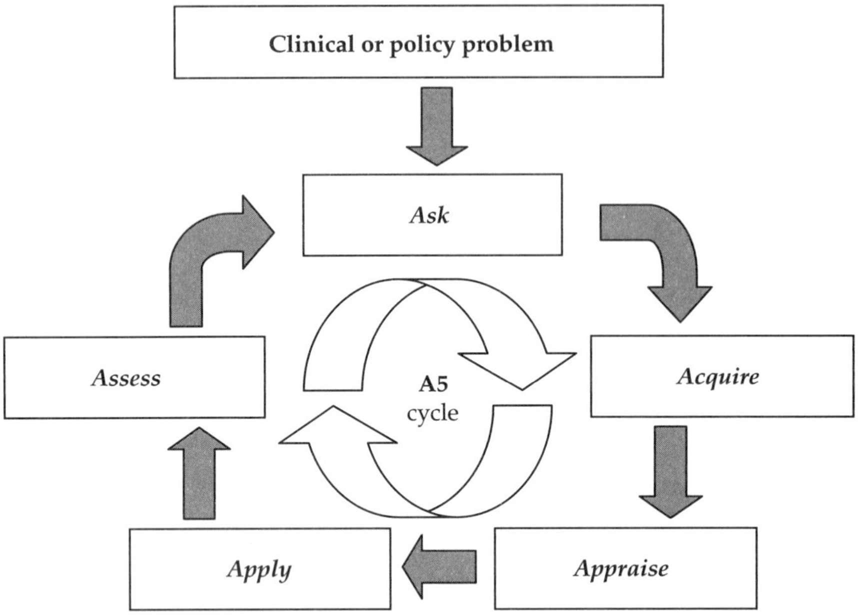

The principles of EBLM comprise five areas of activity relating to the clinical problem or policy:

1. **Asking or formulating the question** that describes the problem.
2. **Acquiring the evidence** that addresses the question.
3. **Appraising the evidence** for relevance and quality.
4. **Applying the knowledge** that is gleaned from the evidence in resolving the problem.
5. **Assessing or auditing the application** to test the robustness of the knowledge and the process of application.

The practical approach to each of these activities will be described in greater detail with examples in Part 2 of this workbook.

Key Concept

Applying the principles of EBLM requires a change from "business as usual." By acquiring and translating high-quality evidence of test effectiveness into an objective assessment of health outcomes, the laboratorian not only becomes a full member of the clinical team but also makes the business case for implementing new diagnostic tools and strategies that can meet clinical needs. The laboratorian thus also has an important role in implementing change.

What Skills Do We Need to Practice EBLM?

In order to undertake EBLM as part of our daily practice it is helpful to be able to acquire the necessary skills and be able to know when to use them most effectively. The table below describes a range of activities that are part of the daily practice of EBLM. Some of these core skills can be developed in Part 2 of this workbook, where you'll work through some examples and have an opportunity to record your own experiences.

Basic EBLM in Day-to-Day Laboratory Practice*

Activity	Skills	Applications
Identifying clinical need	**Formulating answerable questions: PICO**	- What test to use - Designing a study - What does a result mean? - Audit of test usage
Searching for evidence	**Search strategies** **Use of Medline, Embase, etc.**	- Finding all the relevant papers - Is there any evidence?
Reading a paper	**Critical appraisal** **RAMMbo, QUADAS, STEP**	- Are the data relevant to my patient(s)? - Are the data robust?
Reviewing evidence	**Searching the literature** **Critical appraisal** **Meta-analysis**	- Identifying all papers - Ensuring papers (data reported) meet quality criteria - Ensuring statistical analysis is robust
Dissemination, education	**Critically appraised topics (CATs)**	- Keeping up to date
EBLM and laboratory management and policymaking		
Preparing guidelines	**Searching evidence** **Critical appraisal of systematic reviews** **Quality of evidence** **Meta-analysis**	- Is the evidence relevant to my patient(s)? - Is there sufficient evidence? - Is the evidence robust (i.e., to define a guideline)?
Appraising guidelines	**AGREE tool**	- Are the guidelines robust? - Is the guidance reproducible? - Are the guidelines relevant to my patient(s)?
Audit	**Formulating answerable clinical questions**	- Is this test/diagnostic protocol being used properly?

Continued

Basic EBLM in Day-to-Day Laboratory Practice* (Cont'd)

Activity	Skills	Applications
		- Why have the requests for this test risen so steeply? - Is this test being used appropriately? - Is my patient benefiting from use of this test?
Business case for a new test	**Outcomes studies** **Critical appraisal of data** **Economic analysis**	- Will sensitive troponin assays improve outcomes? - Introducing cystatin C as a replacement for creatinine - Introducing urine protein:creatinine ratio to rule out 24-h protein excretion
Policymaking: setting up a new service	**Outcome studies** **Critical appraisal of data** **Economic analysis**	- Initiating a screening program for *Chlamydia* - Devolving chronic disease management to the community
Research skills in EBLM		
Clinical research/developing evidence	**Study design** **Analytical performance** **Diagnostic accuracy studies** **Monitoring studies** **Outcome studies**	- Assessing diagnostic accuracy - Does precision meet clinic need? - Identifying outcomes: use of a test - Launching a new test
Analysis and interpretation of data	**Statistics**	- Accuracy and precision - Does the test improve on pre-test probability?
Reporting evidence/writing a paper	**Writing a paper: STARD**	- Accurate report of study - Meeting quality criteria - Minimizing bias

*The various acronyms are explained later in the text and are defined in Part 3 of this book.

Key Concept

EBLM skills are "transferable": some can be used to research the clinical questions that come up as well as inform day-to-day laboratory management and even help set guidelines and make policy—as from "developing evidence" to "applying evidence."

Pause and Reflect

Consider the skills required to practice EBLM (see table). In which are you strong? (Mark these with a "plus" sign.) Which ones can you strive to improve—or delegate to a team member whose skills are complementary to yours? (Mark these with an "up" arrow.)

After you've completed this workbook, revisit this skills table. What changes have you noticed—and what action steps can you take to get your laboratory/EBLM skills where you'd like them to be?

Where Can We Use EBLM in Our Daily Practice?

Translation of evidence into practice is a crucial part in the practice of EBLM. Evidence can be considered the theoretical component of the practitioner's knowledge base; applying that evidence to solve practical problems is the key to success, especially as measured against patient, clinical user, and provider organization objectives.

One piece of evidence, e.g., from a good quality paper or from a systematic review, can be used in a range of different situations, such as the ones below, and can be used to address issues of interest to different healthcare professionals with different perspectives. (Some of these same scenarios will also be explored in case studies in subsequent sections of this workbook.)

Applications

Clinicians ask what test to use. A clinician may contact you and describe a clinical picture and his/her suspicions as a prelude for requesting advice on what test to use. This may include some of his/her own ideas on which test might be appropriate, a view that may have been shaped by recent articles in the literature or from mailings. The questions will generally be unstructured and you will need to tease out the structure of the question in such a way that it can be addressed—i.e., that you will be able to use the structured question to find an answer, if one exists, from the current literature. Formulating an answerable question is Step 1 (Ask) in practicing EBLM and is addressed in Part 2 of this workbook. Some examples of general questions could include

- Can I use HbA1c for the diagnosis of diabetes?
- I have a 52-year-old man who wants to know if he has prostate cancer. What is the best testing strategy to use?
- Is myoglobin the appropriate test to use for early MI diagnosis?
- Is there a test for patients likely to develop sepsis?

Clinicians wonder how to use a test. Many tests require specific collection conditions and this i... ...tion may not be readily

ac... ...n other situations there may be a

... ...ituations there should be an

... ...e advice that is going to be

... the pre-analytical phase;

... ...igh proportion of

... ...rrect collection tube,

... possible to reconfigure the

... ...tion in order to find the

... ...neral questions could include

- ... ...n measurement?
- ... ...de if I send it from my
- ... a patient who has just ... ...ler to assess his cholesterol
- ... ...ed if I do not collect a
- ... ...at I should collect when

C... ...ng of a specific test r... ...f the result is

u... ...tify the nature of the

pa... why the clinician took a

sa... ...nario when you are the

"d... station. It will also be

im... ...ent, especially to check

for... any respects these

que... ...he patient first

cons... ...nstruct an answerable

ques... ...neral questions could

inclu...

- ...ave just had a potassium result of 5.8 mmol/L on one of my patients who is not symptomatic. Can you explain this?
- I sent a sample in for liver function tests as part of an insurance screen and the bilirubin has come back as 2.0 mg/dL (35 μmol/L). What does it mean?

- Patient X's C-reactive protein (CRP) is 3.5 mg/L. What is her risk of developing coronary artery disease in the next 10 years?
- The glucose measured at bedside is 275 mg/dL (15.3 mmol/L) and the laboratory value measured simultaneously is 210 mg/dL (11.66 mmol/L). Is this variation larger than expected?
- A renal dialysis patient has a cardiac troponin T that is elevated to 0.5 ng/mL but the patient does not have signs and symptoms of myocardial infarction. What is going on?

Clinicians inquire about what decision to make upon receipt of a test result. Many pathologists and laboratorians may see patients as part of a consultative commitment and/or may participate in clinical team meetings, e.g., oncology multidisciplinary team meetings, ward rounds, etc. Others may contribute to a duty rotation dealing with queries that come to the laboratory. In any of these situations a clinician may wish to discuss the decisions following receipt of specific results. Again, it's an "out of the blue" situation! If the respondent is unfamiliar with the patient, it is important to get some background in order to begin the process of formulating the question that is being asked in a way that provides all the information to ensure using the right "evidence" in the response. Some examples of general questions could include

- What should I do when I receive a PSA result of 6.5 ng/mL on a patient who has asked for a PSA test?
- I received a positive result for an antibody test for heparin-induced thrombocytopenia that the technologist said was just barely above the cut-off. Does this slight positivity increase the likelihood that this is a false positive result, such that I can send the patient to surgery without heparin precautions?
- The cardiac troponin is slightly above the cut-off for my emergency department patient. The CK-MB is negative and the patient is doing well; should I send the patient home?
- The B-type natriuretic peptide result is 40 pg/mL (11.6 pmol/L) for my breathless patient. Does this rule out heart failure?

Clinicians request the introduction of a new test. It is not uncommon for clinicians to contact the laboratory after having read a paper, or listened to a lecture, that has featured a new test and to wish to discuss its use in his/her patients. It is also possible that a clinician will come to the laboratory with a problem and ask you if the laboratory service can provide a solution. It is also possible that the laboratory director visits all of the service users on a regular basis to review service quality and experience and assess whether there are any unmet needs. In some of these scenarios the starting point may be fairly academic or research orientated; in others it may be expressing a genuine need. Whatever approach is taken, the starting point for a response must be to define the clinical question or the clinical need. Clearly if there is not an answer available in the literature, then the question can become the basis of a research question and lead to a study. From the laboratorian's point of view, these questions are primarily concerned with the diagnostic performance of a test, or possibly its use in monitoring, and the potential outcome. Some examples of general questions could include

- I have been reading about B-type natriuretic peptide and I think it would be very helpful for managing my treatment of newly diagnosed heart failure. What do you think?
- I have been reading about the soluble transferrin receptor test and I think it would be a better way of assessing iron stores in my dialysis patients than the approach we currently take. What do you think?
- I understand that the serum measurement of HER-2/neu level is increased in a significant proportion of patients with breast cancer at the time of diagnosis of metastatic disease, but who were tissue negative at primary diagnosis. Would this be a good way of detecting metastatic disease?
- Can we have procalcitonin results for our intensive care patients?
- Will the measurement of serum S100 protein improve the detection of recurrent disease in patients with melanoma?

Managers request a business case for the introduction of a new test. At this point the issues move from the potential benefits and risks of introducing the test to the costs of introducing the test, the savings from introducing the test, the area in which those savings will be made, and any changes in clinical practice required to deliver the patient outcomes and the economic benefits. It is implicit in this scenario that managers look for evidence of acceptance of the plan from all of those who are likely to be involved in its delivery! Some examples of general questions could include

- What is the cost to the hospital of introducing a test for B-type natriuretic peptide in the emergency department?
- What are the health economics of introducing intra-operative parathyroid hormone measurement in patients requiring parathyroidectomy?
- What is the value of introducing genotyping for Cytochrome P450 2C9 and Vitamin K Epoxide Reductase Complex Subunit-1 (VKORC1) prior to initial dosing for patients on coumadin (warfarin)?
- What are the benefits from measuring reticulocyte hemoglobin levels in patients with renal failure?
- Will implementation of fetal fibronectin testing allow safe discharge of obstetrics patients admitted for possible contractions related to delivery?

National health policymakers want to introduce a screening program. Approaches to implementing screening programs vary by country and health economy, although there are clear criteria for judging the effectiveness of such a program. These criteria include the availability of a robust test as well as of an effective treatment, and that the benefits outweigh the risks. Some examples of general questions could include the following—and will no doubt have been asked over the years:

- What is the optimal screening program for detection of those carrying a baby with Down syndrome?
- What is the case for screening for *Chlamydia* infection?
- Should we screen for early detection of individuals with type 2 diabetes?
- What is the best approach for screening for early detection of individuals with colon cancer?
- Are we able to screen for men at risk of developing prostate cancer?

A laboratory director requires evidence of method performance and the impact on outcome. Though laboratorians always seek the best quality of analytical performance that can be achieved, there are sometimes cases where questions can arise as to whether this quality is good enough.

In addition, questions arise when choices are available, e.g., when procuring new instrumentation, or when using multiple markers. The challenge is to determine how differing levels of performance, be it in accuracy or precision, impact the health outcomes. Some examples of general questions could include

- Should we be using a blood glucose meter or the glucose module on the blood gas analyzer for maintaining tight glycemic control in patients in the ICU?
- What analytical performance should be the goal when obtaining glucose meters for our patients?
- What precision should we be looking for in each of the methods included in our Down syndrome screening program, and how will variations impact the performance of the final risk score?
- What precision should we be seeking in a B-type natriuretic peptide method to be used for monitoring therapy for patients newly diagnosed with heart failure?
- Can we use a semi-quantitative urine albumin:creatinine ratio using a dipstick test and reader to rule out microalbuminuria in diabetics?

Managers want to change the mode of delivery of care, e.g., move to care of long-term conditions in the community setting. Achieving benefits often requires a change in practice so that those benefits can be delivered. This may include using a test where one had not been available before, using a different test, changing the turnaround time, using POCT, etc.—and any of these options can be suggested by the laboratory director. Alternatively, the clinical service director or manager may come to you with a problem in the hope that you can provide a solution. There are benefits and risks to be considered in relation to both the impact of any change on the quality of care and the clinical outcomes, as well as the economic considerations. Some examples of general questions could include

- Will improving the turn-around time for laboratory investigations in the emergency department reduce the time that patients spend in the emergency department, and in particular the delays that can occur at peak times?
- Will POCT in the emergency department solve some of these problems?
- Will provision of HbA1c results using POCT enable me to shift a significant proportion of my diabetes management into primary care?

- Will provision of intra-operative parathyroid hormone measurements enable me to move parathyroidectomy cases to a day case surgery unit?
- Will pre-admission testing for MRSA reduce the hospital-acquired infection rate?

Managers request an audit of test utilization. Anecdotes abound where the laboratory workload has risen following the publication of a paper, featuring a new test, in a widely read journal. In general, inappropriate testing is shorthand for additional unnecessary testing. However it is also possible that too little testing is undertaken. Strictly speaking, this sort of situation should extend to ensuring that test results are read by the clinician responsible for the care of the patient and that appropriate action is taken. All of these situations come under the broad heading of demand management and performance management. One of the most common tools used—often because it is easy to do—is to compare use of tests between peers. However it is a rather unsophisticated approach and does not enable the laboratorian to ascertain the reasons for differences in laboratory use. Some examples of general questions could include

- Why have the numbers of CRP measurements risen by 20% in the last year?
- We are spending a lot of money on glucose strips. Is there evidence to support the use of self-monitoring of blood glucose in type 2 diabetics?
- Why are liver function tests ordered every day on patients in the ICU?
- What is the optimal frequency for measuring HbA1c in diabetics?
- Is it necessary to order a manual differential count on hospitalized cancer patients more than once a day?

A laboratory director wishes to stop the use of a test. It is often said that while new tests are added to the laboratory repertoire, few are ever dropped. Also, test menus differ between laboratories, and when staff move from one hospital or community to another they invariably request the tests with which they have gained their experience. Some examples of general questions could include

- Why do we still measure gamma glutamyl transferase?
- Why do we still use creatine kinase as a cardiac marker?

- Is there any value in measuring total iron binding capacity as part of the assessment of iron status?
- Do we need to measure total protein as part of the liver function test profile?
- Does osteocalcin have any value as a bone marker?

Key Concept

Often the initial question that you receive from a clinician, manager, healthcare policymaker, or fellow laboratorian is not directly answerable using research and will need to be reformulated. The starting point will always be understanding the issue and asking the question. If this is not done properly, the rest of the process—and the outcome—will be compromised.

Moving from Problems to Solutions

Solving a clinical problem using EBLM is a cyclical process. It begins with generating an answerable question and ends with assessing the process.

Formulating an answerable question from the general questions typically asked by clinicians is the key to initiating and practicing EBLM. This process is addressed in Part 2 Step A1 of this workbook.

Finding the evidence. Now that you know how to formulate the question, you are in a good position to go out and find the evidence. Finding the evidence is about determining whether an answer is already available in the literature, or whether you have to consider developing a study to answer the question. This is covered in Part 2 Step A2 of this book.

Appraising the quality of the evidence. The literature contains evidence of variable quality, so you need to be able to determine whether the results are of good quality in order to have the confidence to develop the answer to the question that was asked in the first place. This is covered in Part 2 Step A3 of this book.

Applying the evidence. Let's assume for the moment that you have found evidence to answer your question and that this evidence is of good quality. Now the fun really starts because you are into one of the most challenging aspects of the laboratorian's practice—changing clinical practice. As we said earlier, there is going to be a change to the "business as usual"—otherwise what's the point! How to apply the evidence is covered in Part 2 Step A4 of this book.

Assessing the process. Once you have applied the evidence, you need to assess—or audit—the process ... not only for the person who asked the question in the first place, but also for YOURSELF. So.... has the change (e.g., from introducing the new test) delivered the outcomes that were expected based on the evidence that you found? Did the EBLM process work efficiently and effectively for you? Part 2 Step A5 of this book will help you to consider these points.

Key Concepts

Acquiring good quality evidence, paying careful attention to the application of evidence, and assessing that process, are keys to achieving better outcomes.

Coming Full Circle: Key Learning Points

Remember the scenarios, presented early in this chapter, about EBLM in the clinical laboratory? You may be interested in how they turned out:

Case 1: Analytical Performance: Assessing Tight Glycemic Control

The director of the hospital's ICU is implementing tight glycemic control for patients on the unit. He asks the ICU's clinical chemist which glucose measurement system he should be using.

The choice lies between providing a rapid central laboratory service or using POCT. The options for POCT amount to either the use of a hand-held patient glucose system or using the glucose module on the benchtop blood gas and electrolyte analyzer.

What do you advise, and why?

What was known: The inter-assay imprecision of the blood gas and electrolyte system glucose channel is about half that of the hand-held blood glucose meter, and there are differences in the calibration (bias) of the two systems, which may have impacted on the choice of sample used.

So the clinical chemist conducted a quick search of PubMed for any papers on tight glycemic control in intensive care patients that looked at the performance of the glucose measurement system. Two papers showed that there were significant discrepancies between using the results obtained from arterial and capillary s[illegible]. This could have led to discrepancies in decisions that w[illegible]n made on the insulin doses.

The clinical chemi[illegible] system should be used as i[illegible]n using arterial sa[illegible]ad been used to deve[illegible]

The key learn[illegible] test may have an impact [illegible]

Literature Sources for This Case

Corstjens AM, Ligtenberg JJ, van der Horst IC, et al. Accuracy and feasibility of point-of-care and continuous blood glucose analysis in critically ill ICU patients. Crit Care 2006;10:R135.

Kanji S, Buffie J, Hutton B, et al. Reliability of point-of-care testing for glucose measurement in critically ill adults. Crit Care Med 2005;33:2778–85.

❖❖❖

Case 2: Nephrology, Cystatin C, and Glomerular Filtration Rate

Your laboratory receives a request from the local nephrologist to start measuring cystatin C, because it appears to provide a better estimate of glomerular filtration rate than serum creatinine. If you were the laboratory director, what would you do?

In this case, the head of the laboratory conducted a search of the literature and found a substantial number of papers comparing the measurement of cystatin C with reference measurements of glomerular filtration rate, e.g., Cr-EDTA clearance, including two meta-analyses. The evidence indicated that cystatin C does correlate better with the reference method for measurement of glomerular filtration rate, and furthermore it may be a better measure in children and elderly individuals. There was also some evidence that cystatin C may be an earlier marker of renal impairment, an early marker of prediabetes and an independent cardiovascular risk factor. However the laboratory director was unable to find any convincing evidence that the use of cystatin C measurement would lead to any improvement in health outcomes.

Somewhat concerned about the difference in cost of providing the test (the cystatin C measurement is an immunoassay whereas the creatinine measurement is a fairly inexpensive colorimetric method), the director decides to present the data on the diagnostic performance of cystatin C to the nephrologist and then ask what clinical problems the cystatin C measurement will be used to address, and what the expected improvements in outcome are likely to be. The nephrologist identifies a couple of areas where he considers the cystatin C measurement to offer benefit over serum creatinine, but that there is no evidence to back up the claim—and so an agreement is reached to embark on the planning of a couple of studies that address the unmet need.

The key learning point is that when considering the introduction of a new test there should be evidence of improved diagnostic performance compared with current practice, and that with the introduction of the new tests there should be some benefit in health outcome.

Literature Sources for This Case

Finney H, Bates CJ, Price CP. Plasma cystatin C determinations in a healthy elderly population. Arch Gerontol Geriatr 1999;29:75–94.

Finney H, Newman DJ, Thakkar H, et al. Reference ranges for plasma cystatin C and creatinine measurements in premature infants, neonates, and older children. Arch Dis Child 2000;82:71–5.

Laterza OF, Price CP, Scott MG. Cystatin C: an improved estimator of glomerular filtration rate? Clin Chem 2002;48:699–707.

Roos JF, Doust J, Tett SE, Kirkpatrick CM. Diagnostic accuracy of cystatin C compared to serum creatinine for the estimation of renal dysfunction in adults and children—a meta-analysis. Clin Biochem 2007;40:383–91.

Zahran A, El-Husseini A, Shoker A. Can cystatin C replace creatinine to estimate glomerular filtration rate? A literature review. Am J Nephrol 2007;27:197–205.

❖❖❖

Case 3. Use of a Test for Monitoring: B-Type Natriuretic Peptide to Guide Therapy in Patients Treated for Heart Failure

A cardiologist visits the laboratory to inquire about providing B-type natriuretic tests in the clinic to help him guide his management of newly diagnosed patients with heart failure. If you were the laboratory director, what would you tell him?

The laboratory director quickly searched the literature and found three randomized controlled trials that looked at using the B-type natriuretic peptide measurement to guide treatment dosing. Two showed benefit; the third did not, having employed a different outcome measure to the first two (the mean beta-blocker dose achieved after three months). A number of papers indicated that the B-type natriuretic peptide measurement was a good prognostic marker for patients being treated for heart failure.

In subsequent discussion with the cardiologist the laboratory director pointed to the limited amount of evidence, and the apparent wide variation in treatment protocols, and offered to support a trial with the cardiologist.

The **key learning points** are that when considering a new test utility the application must take into account the variety of current clinical practice in relation to the breadth of evidence. Furthermore, ensure that the evidence is based on studies that have used the test as part of the decision-making process, and that the outcome measures are appropriate.

Literature Sources for This Case

Beck-da-Silva L, de Bold A, Fraser M, et al. BNP-guided therapy not better than expert's clinical assessment for beta-blocker titration in patients with heart failure. Congest Heart Fail 2005;11:248–53.

Jourdain P, Jondeau G, Funck F, et al. Plasma brain natriuretic peptide-guided therapy to improve outcome in heart failure: the STARS-BNP Multicenter Study. J Am Coll Cardiol 2007;49:1733–9.

Morimoto T, Hayashino Y, Shimbo T, et al. Is B-type natriuretic peptide-guided heart failure management cost-effective? Int J Cardiol 2004;96:177–81.

Troughton RW, Frampton CM, Yandle TG, et al. Treatment of heart failure guided by plasma aminoterminal brain natriuretic peptide (N-BNP) concentrations. Lancet 2000;355:1126–30.

❖❖❖

Case 4. Improving Clinical Practice and Outcomes: POCT for HbA1c in the Ambulatory Clinic and Primary Care

A public health physician from a local HMO writes to the head of the laboratory, indicating he wants to explore the potential benefits of using POCT for HbA1c in the diabetes center clinics. The physician has heard that improved outcomes can be achieved using this approach, and that this approach helps involve patients in the management of their condition. He asks if there is any evidence on the use of POCT for HbA1c. He also broaches the possibility of moving some diabetes care into the primary care setting. The head of the laboratory asks you to deal with the issue. What would you do?

The local clinical chemist remembered that the National Academy of Clinical Biochemistry had recently published its *Laboratory Management Practice Guidelines on Point-of-Care Testing* and so consulted them for guidance on the use of HbA1c in the management of diabetes. She found that there had been three significant papers and one health technology assessment that showed benefit from using POCT. In addition she also learned that patients who know their HbA1c results have better outcomes than those who are unaware of their current values.

She decided to search PubMed for more recent literature. She found an audit of POCT for HbA1c testing over a four-year time period that compared POCT with measurement by a laboratory service. The POCT group showed significant improvement in the HbA1c values, whereas the laboratory-based service showed no improvement. She also found a randomized controlled trial of POCT against a laboratory-based service conducted in primary care that showed no benefit from using POCT, though when she read the discussion section of the paper she found that the primary care physicians did not change their practice and so did not appear to discuss the results with their patients at the time the measurements were made.

In summarizing the information the clinical chemist concluded that discussing the results with the patient at the time of the consultation was important to achieving better outcomes, and that there was a benefit to using POCT.

The **key learning point** is that when providing a test in a different way (e.g., POCT vs. laboratory-based test) it is important to ensure that clinical practice changes to accommodate the change in the approach to test delivery. This applies both in the study design on which the evidence base has been generated, and also to the way in which the test is applied in routine practice.

Literature Sources for This Case

Aarsand AK, Alter D, Frost SJ, et al. Diagnosis and management of diabetes mellitus. In: Nichols, JH, ed. National Academy of Clinical Biochemistry Laboratory Medicine Practice Guidelines: Evidence-based practice for point-of-care testing. Accessed October 15, 2008, at http://www.aacc.org/members/nacb/LMPG/OnlineGuide/PublishedGuidelines/poct/Pages/default.aspx.

Cagliero E, Levina E, Nathan D. Immediate feedback of HbA1c levels improves glycemic control in type 1 and insulin-treated type 2 diabetic patients. Diabetes Care 1999; 22:1785–9.

Grieve R, Beech R, Vincent J, Mazurkiewicz J. Near patient testing in diabetes clinics: appraising the costs and outcomes. Health Technol Ass 1999;3:1–74.

Khunti K, Stone MA, Burden AC, et al. Randomised controlled trial of near-patient testing for glycated haemoglobin in people with type 2 diabetes mellitus. Br J Gen Pract 2006;56:511–7.

Levetan CS, Dawn KR, Robbins DC, Ratner RE. Impact of computer-generated personalized goals on HbA(1c). Diabetes Care 2002;25:2–8.

Miller CD, Barnes CS, Phillips LS, et al. Rapid A1c availability improves clinical decision-making in an urban primary care clinic. Diabetes Care 2003;26:1158–63.

Petersen JR, Finley JB, Okorodudu AO, et al. Effect of point-of-care on maintenance of glycemic control as measured by A1C. Diabetes Care 2007;30:713–5.

Thaler LM, Ziemer DC, Gallina DL, et al. Diabetes in urban African-Americans. XVII. Availability of rapid HbA1c measurements enhances clinical decision-making. Diabetes Care 1999;22:1415–21.

❖❖❖

Case 5. Assessing Operational Needs: POCT in the Emergency Department to Reduce Length of Stay

The chief executive of your hospital is concerned that the recorded times for length of stay for patients attending the emergency department are increasing, especially at peak times. He calls a meeting of the emergency department staff and the directors of the laboratory and imaging departments. Their charge: to find ways of improving triage times throughout the department. If you were the laboratory director, how would you proceed?

The laboratory director conducted a literature search and found a number of papers showing that (1) several studies had looked at POCT for blood gases and electrolytes concluding little improvement in length of stay; (2) when emergency medicine physicians were asked which tests would best assist their decision making, blood gases and electrolytes were not at the top of the list. When the tests identified by the emergency medicine physicians were provided by POCT, there was a significant reduction in the length of stay.

The **key learning point** here is that when offering a test or alternative ways of providing a test, always ask the users of the service what they require.

Literature Sources for This Case

Kendall J, Reeves B, Clancy M. Point of care testing: randomised, controlled trial of clinical outcome. BMJ 1998;316:1052–7.

Lee-Lewandrowski E, Corboy D, Lewandrowski K, et al. Implementation of a point-of-care satellite laboratory in the emergency department of an academic medical center. Impact on test turnaround time and patient emergency department length of stay. Arch Pathol Lab Med 2003;127:456–60.

Murray RP, Leroux M, Sabga E, et al. Effect of point of care testing on length of stay in an adult emergency department. J Emer Med 1999;17:811–4.

Parvin CA, Lo SF, Deuser SM, et al. Impact of point-of-care testing on patients' length of stay in a large emergency department. Clin Chem 1996; 42:711–7.

❖❖❖

Case 6: Choosing and Implementing a Screening Program

A local HMO policymaker is investigating the possibility of implementing a screening program for Chlamydia *infection following reports of an increase in the complications associated with the infection. An initial conversation with the local microbiologist raises the question as to the best screening method to use, with the recommendation that a DNA amplification method would be the best choice. What would you suggest?*

In effect, the clinical microbiologist is being asked to prepare a business case for the introduction of a screening program. A search through the literature using PubMed identified a number of papers, including several on the cost-effectiveness of a screening program. It becomes clear from the papers reviewed that several factors should be taken into account when considering a screening program including (i) the characteristics of the population to be screened, i.e., age and sex,

(ii) the prevalence of the infection, (iii) the number of opportunities for screening, and (iv) the importance of access to partners.

On balance, in the environment relevant to this HMO, the evidence indicated that it would be cost effective to introduce screening, and furthermore that a DNA amplification method would be the method of choice. It was subsequently agreed that the screening program would be implemented. The policymaker sought the cooperation of the microbiologist in developing and implementing the plan, which ensured that appropriate education and training was provided to all health professionals involved in implementing the program.

The key learning points from this case center on ensuring that, when producing a business case, the populations described in the studies match those of the inquirer. It is also critical that the test is shown to be cost-effective and that the implementation strategy is achievable. It is likely in this particular case that evidence may also be available from health technology assessments and programs that have been implemented in other areas or countries.

Literature Sources for this Case

Howell MR, Quinn TC, Brathwaite W, Gaydos CA. Screening women for *chlamydia trachomatis* in family planning clinics: the cost-effectiveness of DNA amplification assays. Sex Transm Dis 1998;25:108–17.

Howell MR, Quinn TC, Gaydos CA. Screening for *chlamydia trachomatis* in asymptomatic women attending family planning clinics. A cost-effectiveness analysis of three strategies. Ann Intern Med 1998;128:277–84.

Hu D, Hook EW 3rd, Goldie SJ. Screening for *chlamydia trachomatis* in women 15 to 29 years of age: a cost-effectiveness analysis. Ann Intern Med 2004;141:501–13.

Norman JE, Wu O, Twaddle S, et al. An evaluation of economics and acceptability of screening for *chlamydia trachomatis* infection, in women attending antenatal, abortion, colposcopy and family planning clinics in Scotland, UK. BJOG 2004;111:1261–8.

Welte R, Kretzschmar M, Leidl R, et al. Cost-effectiveness of screening programs for *chlamydia trachomatis:* a population-based dynamic approach. Sex Transm Dis 2000;27:518–29.

Summary

One of the key jobs of the laboratorian is problem solving. Thus all of the scenarios described here and elsewhere in this workbook have been outlined in the form of a general question that reflects the issue or problem that is troubling the questioner—in other words, ***"how it might be in real life."***

The first stage in the routine practice of EBLM is to recognize the question and to formulate it in a clear, structured way such that you are able to acquire and assess the evidence in order to provide an answer. The starting point will always be understanding the issue and asking the question. If this is not undertaken properly then the rest of the process is compromised ... as will be the outcome.

This introductory chapter has defined and described the key principles of EBLM. It has identified the skills you will need to practice EBLM, and where you might expect to use them.

Many of the examples quoted are based on the direct experience of the authors and that of their colleagues. Several of these cases have been "worked through" the various stages of the EBLM cycle in the following sections of this book and so can be considered as "real-life" examples.

To become proficient in applying EBLM, you must use the principles yourself. In the following chapters we encourage you to document your own learning experience; this will not only help you directly, but also indirectly as you pass on your knowledge to others through teaching and mentoring.

References

1. Sackett DL, Rosenberg WM, Gray JA, et al. Evidence-based medicine: What it is and what it isn't. BMJ 1996;312:71–2.

2. Guyatt G, Rennie D, eds. User's Guide to the Medical Literature. A Manual for Evidence-Based Clinical Practice. Chicago: JAMA and Archive Journals, American Medical Association, 2002:706pp.

3. Glasziou P, Del Mar C, Salisbury J. Evidence-Based Practice Workbook, 2nd ed. Oxford: Blackwell Publishing BMJ Books, 2007:202pp.

4. Del Mar C, Doust J, Glasziou P. Clinical Thinking. Evidence, Communication and Decision-Making. Oxford: Blackwell Publishing BMJ Books, 2006:127pp.

5. Richardson WS, Wilson MC, Nishikawa J, Hayward RS. The well-built clinical question: a key to evidence-based decisions. ACP J Club 1995;123:A12–3.
6. Muir Gray JA. Evidence-based Healthcare: How to Make Health Policy and Management Decisions, 2nd ed. Edinburgh: Churchill Livingstone, 1997:270pp.
7. Price CP, Christenson RH, eds. Evidence-Based Laboratory Medicine: Principles, Practice, and Outcomes, 2nd ed. Washington, DC: AACC Press, 2007:545pp.
8. Sackett DL, Haynes RB. The architecture of diagnostic research. BMJ 2002;324:539–41.
9. Fryback FG, Thornbury JR. The efficacy of diagnostic imaging. Med Decis Making 1991;11:88–94.
10. Deeks J. Assessing outcomes following tests. In: Price CP, Christenson RH, eds. Evidence-Based Laboratory Medicine: Principles, Practice, and Outcomes, 2nd ed. Washington, DC: AACC Press, 2007:95–111.
11. U.S. Department of Health and Human Services. Medicare, Medicaid, and CLIA programs: Regulations implementing the Clinical Laboratory Improvement Amendments of 1988 (CLIA). Final rule. Fed Regist 1992;57:7002–186.
12. Price CP. Evidence-based laboratory medicine: Supporting decision-making. Clin Chem 2000;46:1041–50.
13. Strauss SE, Richardson WS, Glasziou P, Haynes RB. Evidence-Based Medicine. How to Teach and Practice EBM, 3rd ed. Edinburgh: Elsevier Churchill Livingstone, 2005:299pp.
14. The Cochrane Collaboration: the reliable source of evidence in health care. Accessed June 5, 2008, at http://www.cochrane.org.
15. BMJ Clinical Evidence. Accessed June 2, 2008, at http://clinicalevidence.bmj.com/ceweb/index.jsp.

Part 2

Steps in EBLM—The A5 Cycle

STEP A1: ASK—Formulate an Answerable Question

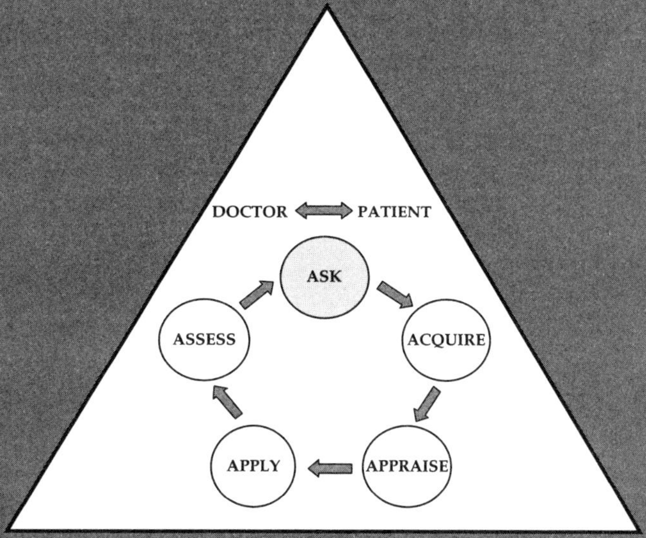

In this chapter

- An overview of the doctor—patient relationship
- Differentiating background and foreground questions
- How good questions help clearly articulate the problem
- The PICO approach
- Derivatives of PICO: prior test, setting, time, change (management)
- Applying PICO to cases (etiology, screening, diagnosis, prognosis, treatment) and perspectives (analytical, operational, economic)
- Opportunities for you to practice and record your own PICOs

The Doctor-Patient Relationship: Putting Questions into Context

The core of clinical medicine is the interaction between the patient and the clinician or other caregiver. Their conversation is basically around a series of questions—to try and resolve the problem. These questions might be general, such as "How are you?", or more specific, such as "How are the tablets helping you?" The patient will also have questions, such as "What do I have?" or "How long do I have?"

Asking questions is one of the most useful tools the clinician has. Responses to these questions can help the clinician develop a diagnosis or an impression of treatment effectiveness. The clinician may then turn to diagnostic tests to refine his reasoning and solve the problem using Bayesian probabilistic reasoning to determine the probability that the patient has a particular condition *(1)*. Time is also an important part of this process—when the symptoms first appeared, when the blood sample was taken, when the tablets were taken, etc.—so time may be an important component of a question.

The question therefore represents the expression of an unresolved problem or clinical need for which a solution is sought. The solution may be aided by an intervention, including the use of a diagnostic test and/or a therapy. The question should be asked in such a way that it deals with the problem at hand, and expressed in such a way that the result can provide a precise and relevant answer *(2)*. All questions therefore require an answer that should lead to a decision being made and an action taken.

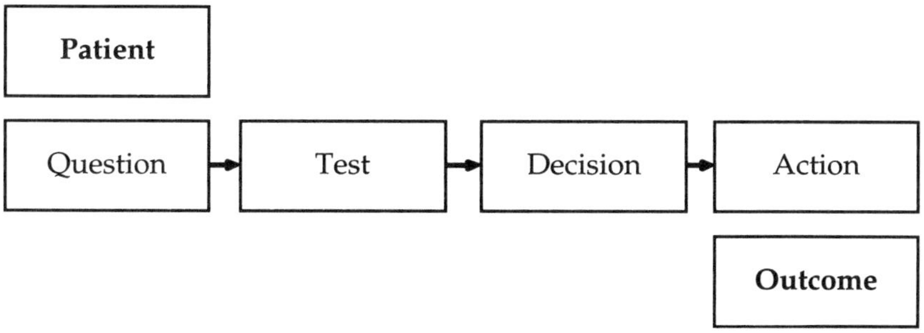

Key Concept

All problems begin with a question. The successful solution to a problem is more likely through the use of a properly structured question.

Differentiating Background and Foreground Questions

Questions can be divided into ***background questions*** and ***foreground questions. Background questions*** are related to the knowledge of the disease that is being considered and of the tests that are being considered. ***Foreground questions*** are more concerned with the application of knowledge and experience in treating the condition and using tests to improve the health outcomes.

The type of background questions you are likely to ask, or be asked, will be clinical or analytical, such as:

- What is rheumatoid arthritis?
- What is responsible for the swelling of joints in rheumatoid arthritis?
- When and why does the serum C-reactive protein (CRP) concentration rise in rheumatoid arthritis?
- What is the analytical specificity of the CRP method?
- What is the precision of the method?
- What is the biological variation of CRP?

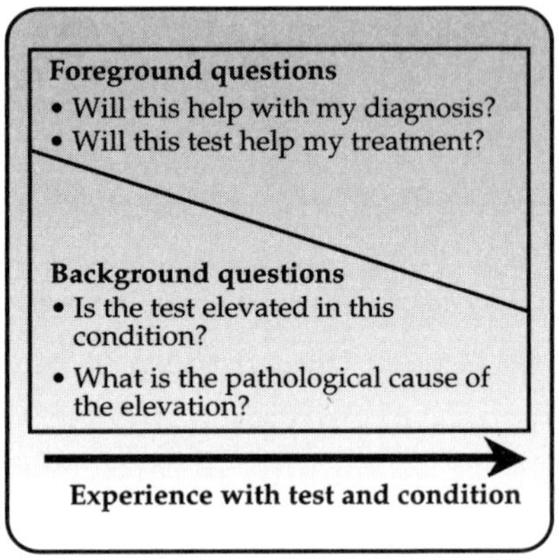

The type of foreground questions you are likely to ask, or be asked, will be on clinical, operational, or economic issues. Here are some examples:

- Will the measurement of CRP be helpful in the diagnosis of rheumatoid arthritis?
- Will CRP be helpful in the management of rheumatoid arthritis?
- Will POCT for CRP help improve health outcomes in the management of rheumatoid arthritis?
- Will regular monitoring of CRP at home help reduce the cost of care associated with managing rheumatoid arthritis?

Differentiating Background & Foreground Q2

Wha ... ourself over the past few

h ... . %

h ... . %

Wha ... ues over the past few

h ... . %

ha ... . %

Write down some examples for future reference:

How Good Questions Help Articulate the Problem

Although the methods for formulating an answerable question were developed to inform clinical decisions on individual patient care, they are equally applicable to the practice of laboratory medicine. You will find that asking a question in a structured way helps to articulate the problem in a clear and precise manner.

In our experience, questions can be used to help solve problems on

- the background to a condition or test—etiology and risk factors
- pre-analytical considerations for tests
- analytical performance of a test
- mode of delivery of a test
- use of tests for screening—diagnostic performance in a screening program
- use of tests in diagnosis—diagnostic performance
- use of tests for prognosis—prognostic performance
- treatment selection—candidacy, minimizing risk, and improving outcomes
- treatment optimization
- treatment compliance
- health economics of testing

In addition, as you will see later, correct formulation of the question is central to literature review and study design in any of the above issues.

The "PICO" Principle

Questions related to patient care are generally composed of four parts:

1. **P**atient—population or problem being addressed
2. **I**ntervention being considered—what test or treatment?
3. **C**omparator or control—what is the intervention of interest going to be compared against?
4. **O**utcome—which can vary depending on the nature of the question

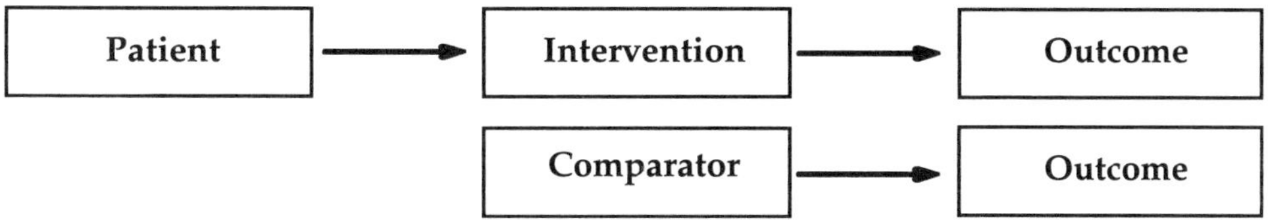

Derivatives of PICO

Prior test. When clinicians try to establish a diagnosis, they have a number of observations that contribute to probabilistic reasoning, beginning with the likelihood of seeing the condition being considered in this particular patient.

The likelihood of a condition will vary according to the patient's other circumstances and characteristics. For example, the prevalence of microalbuminuria is greater in patients with diabetes than in those without; a urinary tract infection is a more likely diagnosis in a patient with positive leukocyte esterase and nitrite urinalysis tests who has a history of urinary tract infections than in a patient without this history.

So, it can be helpful to add another element to the PICO formula, namely **P** for **Prior test**—making it **PPICO.**

When using likelihood ratios and the Fagan nomogram (see Part 3) to judge the performance characteristics of an assay, it is very helpful to use the PPICO approach, as pre-test probability can have a major impact on determining whether adding another test is helpful.

Setting. By setting we mean the place where the patient is seen by the doctor or other healthcare professional, and where the decision is made to employ a test to help make a decision. The setting can be an important determinant of the data-forming part of the evidence to support the use of a test.

Invariably patients with the same condition who present in different settings will reflect different stages in the evolution of the condition. Thus, when a patient begins suffering with chest pain at home, this represents an earlier stage in the evolution of a myocardial infarction than in a patient presenting in the emergency department, and consequently the range of troponin levels found is likely to differ. Consequently, the diagnostic performance of the test in these two "settings" is likely to differ.

Healthcare systems differ in their planning and organization, with differing contributions being made by primary, secondary, and tertiary care. This may then reflect in the characteristics of patients presenting in the different settings—and thus, again, the severity of the condition at presentation may differ. Consequently, the range of results that are found in these differing populations of patients will also vary.

The type of healthcare system may extend to organization within a system. Thus, one might expect to find differences in the quality of care provided for patients with long-term conditions depending on whether an integrated program of care is provided, and the effectiveness of this program.

Remember, also, that the "setting" can span a range from the home, workplace, or leisure place, through to highly sophisticated healthcare provider organizations.

This gives us the variant PICOS; it may be used more frequently than you, at first, think!

Time. Time can be a very important consideration:

- Some diagnoses are only made by observing the patient to see how symptoms develop, or the effect of a treatment.
- Time might be an important factor in determining the meaning of a particular result. For example, was the digoxin sample taken at the right time? When was the troponin sample taken?
- Time might be important when conducting a prognostic accuracy study, such as monitoring cardiac events for only 30 days when assessing the potential prognostic meaning of a very small increase in a troponin value.

For these reasons it may be helpful, in certain circumstances, to add a further element to the PICO formula, namely **T** for **Time**—making it **PICOT** *(3)*.

Change (management). Change in this context is used to describe what would happen if a test were used to make a decision, compared with if the test were not used. It could equally apply when considering a change in the mode of delivery, e.g., POCT, and when considering the impact of a test result on an outcome.

A test result is of no value unless a decision is made upon receipt of the result and some action taken if an improved outcome is expected. In this case, a change in the patient management occurs, a change necessary to achieve an improved outcome. Similarly, if a new test is introduced it will lead to a change in practice if the expected improvement in outcome is to be achieved. The introduction of POCT will involve a change in practice, for example, if the expected benefit is to be delivered.

Change (management) may be particularly challenging when there is a change in "setting."

Many studies in the literature cite instances where tests were ordered but no action was taken on the results. How can you then expect any improvement in outcome? For these reasons, it may be helpful in such circumstances to add a further element to the PICO formula, namely **C** for **Change (management)**—making it **PICCO.**

Key Concept

All questions need to follow the core of the PICO principle. As you will see later in this workbook, it can be helpful to add more elements when formulating your question.

Pause and Reflect

Rate your current understanding of the following based on a scale of 1 (poor) to 10 (excellent):

(i) the difference between background and foreground questions ....

(ii) the different types of questions, e.g., diagnostic accuracy, treatment, etc. ....

(iii) how questions help clearly articulate the problem ....

(iv) the P of PICO ....

(v) the I of PICO ....

(vi) the C of PICO ....

(vii) the O of PICO ....

(viii) when to use PPICO ....

(ix) when to use PICOS ....

(x) when to use PICOT ....

(xi) when to use PICCO ....

Is there anything in particular that you are struggling with? Make a note and come back to it at the end of this section of the workbook.

....

....

....

....

....

....

....

....

....

....

....

....

....

Types of questions may include:

- etiology and risk factors
- pre-analytical considerations
- analytical performance of a test
- mode of delivery of a test
- diagnostic performance in a screening program
- diagnostic performance in other situations
- prognostic performance
- treatment selection—candidacy, minimizing risk, and improving outcomes
- treatment optimization
- treatment compliance
- health economics of testing

Constructing PICO Questions

The remainder of this section explores a wide range of clinical scenarios (etiology, screening, diagnosis, prognosis, treatment) and perspectives (analytical, operational, and economic). Each scenario or perspective presents background on "typical" questions that might be asked, then lists a number of case studies for each. In each case, an unstructured question has been asked.

The PICO approach is then presented and the question restated. After several of these examples, you will practice this skill yourself. Remember that you can always add the additional elements—P for Prior test, S for Setting, T for Time, or C for Change. Good luck!

Key Concept

This is not an "exact science" and you may struggle to fit all of your questions rigidly into the framework we are proposing. Sometimes it may not be possible to find a comparator to include in your PICO. You may also find that you are using the additional elements of the PICO derivatives, P, S, T, and C, in PPICO, PICOS, PICOT, and PICCO, in different ways.

It doesn't matter! Because, just by going through this approach you will bring greater clarity to the questions you are being asked, or are asking yourself.

In so doing we think you will find it easier to develop more structured questions–the kinds of questions at the heart of solving any clinical problem.

Etiology, Risk Factors, and Prevalence

Questions about etiology, risk factors, and prevalence usually address what might be called the "basic science" of the disease and of the tests that might be used to help the clinician manage a patient. In clinical practice, these questions tend to focus on the harms associated with an intervention, although in a laboratory investigation they may be more about understanding what causes a change in an analyte concentration (possibly an unexpected or unexplained change) or the frequency of a change in the analyte concentration in a patient with a certain condition. Some of these questions may be pre-analytical (addressed later).

In cases where a derivative of the PICO formula is helpful, we have included it.

Case 1. *A 34-year-old woman who has been running five miles every day for six weeks as part of her preparation for a local fundraising event collapses after one of these runs, and is admitted to the hospital complaining of chest pains. No ECG changes were found, but a serum troponin I measurement reveals a level of 0.02 ng/L (upper reference interval 0.01 ng/L). The admitting physician wishes to know if sustained physical exercise can increase the serum troponin level.*

P: women

I: sustained physical exercise

C: normal lifestyle exercise

O: serum troponin level

Question: In women around 35 years of age, will sustained physical exercise, such as running five miles daily, increase the serum troponin level, compared with women who only undertake normal lifestyle exercise?

Case 2. *A 42-year-old woman with a history of renal impairment is admitted to the emergency department with symptoms of breathlessness. She is found to have a B-type natriuretic peptide (BNP) level of 385 pg/mL and a serum creatinine of 3.7 mg/dL (327 µmol/L), eGFR = 14 mL · minute*$^{-1}$ · $(1.73\ m^2)^{-1}$.

P: women with renal impairment

I: BNP measurement

C: women with normal renal function

O: BNP concentration

Question: Are BNP concentrations increased in women with renal impairment compared to women of similar age with normal renal function (i.e. eGFR >60 mL · minute^{-1} · (1.73 m^2)$^{-1}$)?

Case 3. *At a routine health screening, a male is found to have a total cholesterol of 254 mg/dL (6.5 mmol/L) and his primary care physician prescribes a statin. However, the physician has heard that patients on statins may develop a myositis and myopathy and he wants to know over what period he should monitor the patient.*

P: males on statins having muscle pains

I: creatine kinase

C: males on statins having no muscle pain

O: creatine kinase

T: change in concentrations over time

Question: In men taking statins as treatment for elevated serum cholesterol, at what time will an elevation of the serum creatine kinase that indicates myositis or myopathy most likely be observed?

Now You Try It

Read the case below. Apply the PICO principle. Then develop a search question just as in the examples above. You can check your answers in the box below.

This is the first step in practicing formulating questions that will allow you to search the literature for the inquirer and provide the background evidence that enables you to give informed advice.

Case 4. *A 50-year-old man asks for a prostate specific antigen (PSA) measurement as part of his routine health screen and the result comes back as 5.5 μg/L. He visits his primary care physician and inquires about the likelihood of having prostate cancer. The primary care physician contacts the laboratory asking about age-related reference ranges and what advice he should give his patient.*

Remember the PICO variants: "P" for "prior test," "S" for "setting," "T" for "time," and "C" for "change" (management). Are any of them appropriate here? For example, there is specific guidance offered to primary care physicians in this situation.

P: ....

I: ....

C: ....

O: ....

Question:

....

....

Possible Answers

P: men, ages 40 to 50 years, with no history of prostate cancer

I: serum PSA

C: men, ages 30 to 40 years, and 50 to 60 years and above, with no history of prostate cancer

O: serum PSA reference ranges by decade

Question: What are the reference ranges for serum PSA by decade in men ages 30 to 70 years?

P: men 50 years of age attending a health screen and found to have a serum PSA of 5.5 μg/L

I: serum PSA

C: men, ages 45 to 55 years, with no history of prostate cancer

O: likelihood of having prostate cancer

Question: What is the likelihood of a man of 50 years of age attending a health screen (and presumably with no symptoms) having prostate cancer?

Your Own Cases

Choose two cases in your institution that have come up in your laboratory practice. List them here. Then practice applying the PICO principle to these cases.

Remember to think about the PICO variants. If you choose to use one, or more, of them, then highlight with a note.

Case 5. ....

....

P: ....

I: ....

C: ....

O: ....

Question:

....

....

Case 6. ....

....

P: ....

I: ....

C: ....

O: ....

Question:

....

....

Screening

Screening questions deal with diagnostic accuracy. A screening test will only be of practical value if there is an effective treatment.

The benefits and risks of screening take into account both the test used to screen for the condition and the treatment applied. Screening can however be considered at a societal level, e.g., for population screening, or for use in specific clinical situations.

Case 1. *The local specialists in diabetes are considering introduction of regular annual tests for urine albumin:creatinine ratio in their diabetic population for the early detection of renal nephropathy. They contact the laboratory to obtain the evidence on which to build their case.*

P: patients with type 1 or type 2 diabetes

I: annual random urine albumin:creatinine ratio measurements

C: no testing unless clinically indicated

O: renal impairment

Question: In patients with type 1 or type 2 diabetes, will the introduction of annual urine albumin:creatinine measurement lead to earlier detection of renal impairment?

> A true screening question would link the detection of increased albumin excretion with the initiation of treatment, compared with treatment only initiated according to the current standard of care—the outcome being a reduction in the rate of onset of renal failure and death due to renal failure.

❖❖❖

Case 2. *A local public health physician asks this question: Is screening with fecal occult blood improved by using an immunochemical confirmatory test prior to referral for colonoscopy for the early detection of significant colon neoplasia?*

P: men and women over the age of 50

I: use of reflex to a second (immunochemical) test for all samples that are positive for the guaiac test for fecal occult blood as part of a screening program

C: use of only the guaiac test in the screening program

O: reduction in false positives referred for colonoscopy

> A true screening question would link the detection of significant colon neoplasia using the reflex testing approach with the implementation of treatment, compared with the current screening program pathway, the outcome being a reduction in morbidity and mortality. It would also be possible to pose an economic question looking at the cost benefit of the new approach.

Question: Will adding an immunochemical test for all samples found to be positive using the guaiac test for fecal occult blood improve efficiency of detection of patients with significant colon neoplasia?

❖❖❖

Case 3. *A local public health physician is concerned about the increasing prevalence of type 2 diabetes and its complications. He seeks advice as to whether there is any evidence to support the introduction of screening, with a plan to make such a service available in the local community pharmacy. He notes that several guidelines suggest such measurements be made with an analytical system conforming to laboratory standard performance.*

P: males and females considered to be at risk of developing type 2 diabetes

I: measurement of the fasting blood sugar available in the community pharmacy using an analytical system conforming to laboratory standard performance

C: no testing available other than when clinically indicated

O: detection of patients with type 2 diabetes in the local community

> A true screening question would compare the detection of type 2 diabetes, with confirmation using a laboratory test, to the current practice of detecting and making a diagnosis of type 2 diabetes. It assumes that treatment to manage the diabetes would be implemented and the outcome would be an improvement in mortality associated with the disease. It would also be possible to pose an economic question looking at the cost benefit of screening for type 2 diabetes.

Question: Will screening with a fasting blood sugar measurement, initially available in the community pharmacy, lead to the diagnosis of more patients with type 2 diabetes than at present?

❖❖❖

Now You Try It

Read the case below. Apply the PICO principle. Then develop a search question just as in the examples above. You can check your answers in the box below.

Case 4. *A 50-year-old man visits his primary care physician. He wants to be screened for prostate cancer using the PSA test. The primary care physician phones the laboratory for the latest advice on the use of this test for screening purposes.*

P: ....

I: ....

C: ....

O: ....

Question:

....

....

❖❖❖

Possible Answers

P: men of 50 years of age

I: screening with serum PSA

C: no testing unless clinically indicated

O: prostate cancer

Question: Will screening with serum PSA in men of 50 years of age lead to earlier detection of prostate cancer?

P: men of 50 years of age

I: screening with serum PSA

C: no testing unless clinically indicated

O: mortality

Question: Will screening with serum PSA in men of 50 years of age lead to a reduction in the number of deaths due to prostate cancer?

Your Own Cases

Choose two cases in your own institution that have come up in your laboratory practice. List them here. Then practice applying the PICO principles to these cases.

> Remember to think about the PICO variants. If you choose to use one, or more, of them, then highlight with a note.

Case 5. ....

....

P: ....

I: ....

C: ....

O: ....

Question:

....

....

❖❖❖

Case 6. ....

....

P: ....

I: ....

C: ....

O: ....

Question:

....

....

❖❖❖

Diagnosis

Diagnostic questions deal with the diagnostic accuracy of a test in a range of patient groups and differing situations, compared with other tests that might be available to answer the same clinical question.

In the case of diagnostic accuracy, the outcome (O) is the diagnosis made by the gold standard method.

The range of patient groups may include males and females, children or adults, patients presenting at different stages of the development of their symptoms or of the disease. Ideally the comparison test will be the definitive test, often called the "gold standard test," although it may not always be a test that can be used in a routine situation. In this latter case, one might be looking to see if a new test is better than the test in current use.

If there is no agreed upon diagnostic test available, then the final diagnosis may only be made at a later date as the condition evolves, or at the time of death using post mortem examination.

Case 1. *The consultant microbiologist is concerned about the number of urines being sent from primary care for microscopy, culture, and sensitivity quoting a suspicion of "urinary tract infection." He has read the literature and believes that using a dipstick test for urinalysis might be helpful to either rule in or rule out a diagnosis, thereby reducing the number of urines that would be sent to the laboratory if the initial test were undertaken in primary care.*

Note that the setting is specifically mentioned in this question, and is covered in the "P" element of the question. When searching for evidence, it might be a good idea to use the "S" variant of the PICO to emphasize this point.

P: patients presenting to primary care with symptoms suggestive of a urinary tract infection

I: dipstick urinalysis for leukocyte esterase and nitrite

C: laboratory test for microscopy, culture, and sensitivity

O: urinary tract infection

Question: In patients presenting to primary care with symptoms suggestive of a urinary tract infection, can a dipstick urinalysis test for leukocyte esterase and nitrite be used to reliably rule in or rule out a diagnosis of urinary tract infection and thereby reduce the number of urines that have to be sent to the laboratory for microscopy, culture, and sensitivity?

❖❖❖

Case 2. *A 75-year-old Caucasian man is admitted to the emergency department in acute distress. Upon examination, his chief complaint is dyspnea, which has worsened over the past 12 hours. Further examination reveals rales but no apparent jugular venous distension or edema. An electrocardiogram shows no evidence of cardiac ischemia. The patient's history indicates hypertension, chronic obstructive airways disease, and smoking for the past 50 years. The attending physician suspects that the patient may have acute congestive heart failure and asks if a BNP test is an appropriate test to request.*

P: men presenting with dyspnea and risk factors to the emergency department

I: plasma BNP measurement

C: independent opinion of two cardiologists

O: acute congestive heart failure

> You may want to think of a prior test here—which could be a symptom, such as dyspnea—and consider the performance with and without dyspnea, i.e., the use in symptomatic vs. asymptomatic patients.

Question: What is the diagnostic performance of plasma BNP for the diagnosis of acute congestive cardiac failure in a 75-year-old man with dyspnea and risk factors presenting to the emergency department compared with the accepted gold standard diagnosis provided by the independent opinions of two cardiologists?

> If you take away the dyspnea, and the presentation is less acute, then it may be more important to identify the setting more specifically. You may want to differentiate those patients who present to primary care from those who present to secondary care.

❖❖❖

Case 3. *A nephrologist wants to find a more reliable method for assessing iron status in patients with chronic renal failure treated with iron therapy. He contacts the laboratory to inquire about the use of a new test for reticulocyte hemoglobin content.*

P: patients with chronic renal failure

I: measurement of the reticulocyte hemoglobin content

C: bone marrow iron stores

O: iron status

Question: In patients with chronic renal failure treated with iron therapy, does the measurement of reticulocyte hemoglobin content provide a reliable means of assessing iron status compared with the bone marrow iron store assessment? (*A shorthand version of this question could be "What is the diagnostic performance of the reticulocyte hemoglobin content for the assessment of iron status in patients with chronic renal failure on iron therapy?"*)

❖❖❖

Now You Try It

Read the case below. Apply the PICO principle. Then develop a search question just as in the examples above. You can check your answers in the box below.

Case 4. *A consultant nephrologist emails the clinical chemist and tells her that he has read a number of articles about the measurement of cystatin C in patients with renal failure. He wonders whether it would be a more helpful test than serum creatinine for detecting early changes in glomerular filtration rate associated with a rejection episode in patients following a kidney transplant.*

P: ....

I: ....

C: ....

O: ....

Question:

....

....

❖❖❖

Possible Answers

P: patients following kidney transplant who develop a rejection episode

I: serum cystatin C

C: serum creatinine

O: change in concentrations after operation

Question: Is there any evidence to indicate that the serum cystatin C rises ahead of the serum creatinine in patients following a kidney transplant who subsequently develop a rejection episode?

P: patients following kidney transplant who develop a rejection episode

I: serum cystatin C

C: serum creatinine

O: diagnostic accuracy against a reference method for glomerular filtration rate

Question: Is there any evidence to indicate that the serum cystatin C is a better indicator of the glomerular filtration rate than serum creatinine in patients following a kidney transplant who subsequently develop a rejection episode?

Your Own Cases

Choose two cases in your own institution that have come up in your laboratory practice. List them here. Then practice applying the PICO principle in these cases.

> Remember to think about the PICO variants. If you choose to use one, or more, of them, then highlight with a note.

Case 5. ....

....

P: ....

I: ....

C: ....

O: ....

Question:

....

....

❖❖❖

Case 6. ....

....

P: ....

I: ....

C: ....

O: ....

Question:

....

....

❖❖❖

Prognosis

Prognostic (or prediction) questions are about determining the likelihood of a particular outcome for a population with specific changes observed in the results of laboratory investigations such as the likelihood of a person with an increased serum high-sensitivity CRP level developing an acute coronary syndrome.

Note that prognostic information is frequently of modest value unless the information can be linked to effective management of the patient.

Case 1. *A consultant nephrologist observes a small increase of the troponin T level in a patient with Stage 5 chronic kidney disease. This increase persists over several weeks while measurements are made. The nephrologist wishes to know if these changes have any prognostic significance.*

P: patients with chronic kidney disease

I: serum troponin T level

C: none*

O: cardiac event, e.g., myocardial infarction or cardiac related death

T: within twelve-month follow-up period**

Question: In patients with chronic renal failure, in the presence of an increased circulating level of troponin T, what is likely to predict a future cardiac event?

> * In some situations there is no need for a comparator as you are looking for the relationship between the intervention (I)—in this case an elevation of the serum troponin—and the outcome (O)—a cardiac event.
>
> ** Time is often assessed in the critical appraisal of prognostic studies because the use of short follow-up periods may not be adequate in detecting the risk of a poor outcome.

❖❖❖

Case 2. *An oncologist reads about a new "genetic" test that can predict the likelihood of a patient diagnosed with breast cancer suffering a recurrence. He contacts his colleague in anatomical pathology to find out the level of the evidence to support the claim.*

P: women diagnosed with breast cancer

I: tissue expression of a panel of genes

C: grading of cancer made at diagnosis based on histology, tumor size, etc.

O: recurrence of disease

T: six-month follow-up period

Question: How well can the expression of a panel of genes in the primary tumor at the time of diagnosis in a woman with breast cancer predict the likelihood of recurrence of disease?

❖❖❖

Case 3. *It has been shown that the urinary albumin:creatinine ratio increases in patients admitted to the intensive care unit (ICU) and furthermore that the increase is a good predictor of mortality. The intensive care specialists want to know how the prognostic performance compares with clinical observation and mortality scores such as the APACHE and SOFA scores.*

P: patients admitted to the ICU

I: measurement of the urinary albumin:creatinine ratio

C: APACHE and SOFA scores

O: ICU mortality

T: during ICU stay and post-discharge period

Question: What is the prognostic performance of the urinary albumin: creatinine ratio on admission to the ICU when compared with current clinical practice using indices such as the APACHE and SOFA scores? *(You may wish to differentiate between the ICU stay and the post-discharge periods.)*

❖❖❖

Now You Try It

Read the case below. Apply the PICO principle. Then develop a search question just as in the examples above. You can check your answers in the box.

Case 4. *It has been demonstrated that aberrations of DNA methylation are one of the most consistent epigenetic changes in human cancers. Human cancers generally show widespread DNA hypomethylation accompanied by specific regions of hypermethylation. The implication is that the assessment of the methylation status of specific DNA markers might provide a useful prognostic tool in oncology.*

P: ....

I: ....

C: ....

O: ....

T: ....

Question:

....

....

❖❖❖

Note to the reader: This is a very broad question as we don't know, at this point, whether the observation is applicable in all cancers. Furthermore we don't know whether the specific DNA markers are unique to each type of cancer.

Suggested Answer

P: patients diagnosed with a particular form of cancer

I: methylation status of a defined set of DNA markers

C: none

O: mortality

T: twelve months after testing

Question: Does the methylation status of a defined set of DNA markers provide prognostic information in patients with defined cancers?

This question could therefore be formulated for both types of cancer and methylation status of defined DNA markers.

Your Own Cases

Choose two cases in your own institution that have come up in your laboratory practice. List them here. Then practice applying the PICO principle to these cases.

Remember to think about the PICO variants. If you choose to use one, or more, of them, then highlight with a note.

Case 5. ....

....

P: ....

I: ....

C: ....

O: ....

T: ....

Question:

....

....

❖❖❖

Case 6. ....

....

P: ....

I: ....

C: ....

O: ....

T: ....

Question:

....

....

❖❖❖

Treatment

Many diagnostic questions are then followed by a range of treatment questions that may include

(a) candidacy for a particular drug,
(b) assessing likely responsiveness and risk of harm associated with inappropriate dosage,
(c) assessing efficacy and need to change dose of treatment, and
(d) assessing efficacy and compliance with treatment.

Treatment may also include education and training, patient counseling, and guidance on lifestyle changes.

> Remember, with treatment the outcome will be based on the use of the test and the treatment.

> Remember, adding a test in these situations is likely to introduce a change in practice, and so including the "C" variant of the PICO formula could be important—to ensure that the result was actually used in the decision-making process.

Case 1. *An oncologist wishes to introduce a new cancer drug that targets a specific cell surface antigen. He believes that from the experience gained with Herceptin that it will be necessary to test for the presence of the cell surface antigen before deciding whether to prescribe this new treatment. He asks his colleague in anatomical pathology to determine whether there is any evidence for this supposition, and the degree of treatment benefit in those found to express an increased amount of the cell surface antigen in the tumor tissue compared with those who do not.*

P: patients with breast cancer treated with drug

I: increased expression of cell surface antigen expression in primary tumor tissue

C: normal expression of cell surface antigen

O: morbidity and mortality

> You could add a "T" component to define a follow-up period—which could then be used to inform advice on improved life expectancy.

Question: In patients with breast cancer, will the presence of increased expression of the target cell surface antigen in the primary tumor tissue identify those patients who are likely to benefit from treatment with the new drug?

❖❖❖

Case 2. *A gastroenterologist is asked to prepare the local guidelines for the use of azothioprene in the treatment of inflammatory bowel disease. He recalls a case report in which a patient who was given azothioprene suffered a major hematological crisis, which was subsequently thought to be due to a deficiency of the enzyme thiopurine methyl transferase. He asks the local hematologist for advice on the use of azothioprene in patients with this enzyme deficiency with respect to minimizing the risk of hematological crises.*

P: patients with inflammatory bowel disease

I: guiding use of azothioprene on the basis of an assessment of thiopurine methyl transferase status

C: no assessment of thiopurine methyl transferase status and current standard of care

O: morbidity and mortality

Question: Does the guidance of azothioprene dosage based on a patient's thiopurine methyl transferase status reduce the risk of hematological crises in patients with inflammatory bowel disease?

❖❖❖

Case 3. *A primary care physician has read a couple of editorials that call into question the use of self-monitoring blood glucose in the management of type 2 diabetes. She phones the local clinical chemist to ask about the latest evidence on monitoring blood glucose.*

> Note that HbA1c is used here as a surrogate outcome marker. Increased concentrations are associated with poorer outcomes, i.e., mortality and morbidity—and hence earlier onset of complications.

P: patients with type 2 diabetes

I: self-monitoring of blood glucose as part of an integrated package of care

C: no self-monitoring of blood glucose

C (change management): adjust dosage according to thiopurine methyl transferase status

O: HbA1c concentration

Question: Does the inclusion of self-monitoring of blood glucose as part of an integrated package of care in the management of type 2 diabetes lead to better glycemic control (and by implication) a reduction in the rate of onset of complications?

❖❖❖

Now You Try It

Read the case below. Apply the PICO principle. Then develop a search question just as in the examples above. You can check your answers in the box below.

> Remember to think about the PICO variants.

Case 4. *A cardiologist asks the laboratory to offer the measurement of BNP in order to manage his patients newly diagnosed with heart failure. As part of the business case to justify introducing the test for this application the clinical chemist undertakes a literature review.*

P: ....

I: ....

C: ....

C (change management): ....

O: ....

Question:

....

....

❖❖❖

Possible Answers

P: patients with newly diagnosed heart failure

I: monitoring with plasma BNP measurement

C: current practice (which may be based on signs, symptoms, weight, etc.)

O: achievement of target BNP value

Question: Will the use of BNP measurement to guide treatment in patients with newly diagnosed heart failure lead to more patients achieving a target BNP value compared with current practice?

P: patients with newly diagnosed heart failure

I: monitoring with plasma BNP measurement

C: current practice (which may be based on signs, symptoms, weight, etc.)

O: cardiac-related events

Question: Will the use of BNP measurement to guide treatment in patients with newly diagnosed heart failure lead to a reduction in cardiac-related events, e.g., worsening heart failure, cardiac-related death?

P: patients with newly diagnosed heart failure

I: monitoring with plasma BNP measurement

C: current practice (which may be based on signs, symptoms, weight, etc.)

O: cardiac-related hospitalization, either to ambulatory care or full admission

Question: Will the use of BNP measurement to guide treatment in patients with newly diagnosed heart failure lead to a reduction in hospital visits (either ambulatory care or full admissions)?

Your Own Cases

Choose two cases in your own institution that have come up in your laboratory practice. List them here. Then practice applying the PICO principle to these cases.

Remember to think about the PICO variants. If you choose to use one, or more, of them, then highlight with a note.

Case 5. ....

....

P: ....

I: ....

C: ....

O: ....

Question:

....

....

❖❖❖

Case 6. ....

....

P: ....

I: ....

C: ....

O: ....

Question:

....

....

❖❖❖

Analytical

> Remember, you are thinking about the impact of aspects of analytical performance on the outcome—for the patient, for the clinician, for the provider organization, for the payer.

A number of questions may arise with respect to the choice of analytical method or platform, and every effort is made to achieve the highest quality of analytical performance. However, from time to time issues might arise where a choice exists between methods offering differing levels of analytical performance but having other advantages—e.g., cost, a faster turn-around, or availability of a particular test on a chosen platform being not as good as that on an alternative platform. In addition, a range of pre- and post-analytical issues may impact the effectiveness of a particular test, e.g., the biological variation of an analyte.

Case 1. *The director of the ICU is planning to introduce glucose monitoring to achieve better glycemic control, because it improves morbidity and mortality for patients on the unit. She asks the clinical chemist if the analytical performance (imprecision and bias) of a handheld glucose meter will be adequate to achieve these goals, or whether they should invest in a blood gas and electrolyte analyzer with a glucose electrode (she understands this system offers better analytical performance).*

P: patients in the ICU under a tight glycemic control regime

I: blood glucose measured with a handheld glucose meter

C: blood glucose measured with a blood gas analyzer glucose electrode

O: morbidity and mortality

Question: Will the use of a more accurate and precise glucose measurement system lead to better outcomes when seeking to improve glycemic control in patients in the ICU?*

> * This question could also be posed to address the health economics of using the better test.

❖❖❖

Case 2. *An emergency medicine physician is considering the use of a POCT device for the rapid measurement of troponin in patients admitted with chest pain. He seeks advice as to whether he will gain the same quality of information for risk stratification, and thus subsequent triage, compared with the use of a central laboratory test.*

P: patients presenting to the emergency department with chest pain

I: POCT for troponin

C: central laboratory testing for troponin

O: cardiac event

T: over two-year follow-up period

Question: Will the use of POCT for troponin measurement give the same quality of risk stratification (and by implication the guidance for subsequent triage) compared with a central laboratory measurement?

❖❖❖

Case 3. *A public health policymaker has reviewed the literature on the tests available for screening for Down syndrome and wishes to understand how the choice of different markers, the combination of markers, and the choice of risk calculation algorithm, impacts the performance of a screening program.*

P: pregnant women being screened for carrying a fetus with Down syndrome

I: individual risk calculation algorithms

C: risk calculation by conventional means or alternate algorithms

O: detection of Down syndrome

Question: Does the choice of risk calculation algorithm have an impact on the performance of a Down syndrome screening program?

❖❖❖

Now You Try It

Read the case below. Apply the PICO principle. Then develop a search question just as in the examples above. You can check your answers in the box below.

Case 4. *A prostate risk management program is advocating the use of an assay for PSA that meets certain quality criteria linked with the analytical specificity, and the calibration of the assay. Unfortunately the current assay used in the laboratory does not meet the criteria—so the clinical chemist is asked to check the literature to determine the impact of not meeting these criteria on clinical outcomes. This information will be used to build a business case for complying with the criteria using an alternative analytical platform.*

P: ....

I: ....

C: ....

O: ....

Question:

....

....

❖❖❖

Possible Answers

P: men receiving serum PSA tests as part of a prostate cancer risk management program

I: serum PSA test meeting the agreed quality criteria with respect to accuracy

C: serum PSA test not meeting agreed quality criteria with respect to accuracy

O: unnecessary biopsies avoided and cancers detected

Question: Does the use of a serum PSA test that meets agreed quality criteria with respect to accuracy lead to improved performance of the test (through avoidance of unnecessary biopsies as well as detecting more cancers)?

This is a difficult question to answer as it can only be answered in a practical manner using modeling. So an alternative answer might be this:

P: men receiving serum PSA tests as part of a prostate cancer risk management program

I: variation in accuracy and precision of serum PSA test

C: none

O: unnecessary biopsies avoided and cancers detected

Question: Will variation in the accuracy and precision of a serum PSA test lead to differences in the number of unnecessary biopsies and cancers detected?

Your Own Cases

Choose two cases in your own institution that have come up in your laboratory practice. List them here. Then practice applying the PICO principle to these cases.

Will PICO variants be relevant to any of your cases here? If you choose to use one, or more, of them, then highlight with a note.

Case 5. ....

....

P: ....

I: ....

C: ....

O: ....

Question:

....

....

❖❖❖

Case 6. ....

....

P: ....

I: ....

C: ....

O: ....

Question:

....

....

❖❖❖

Operational

Operational issues in laboratory medicine invariably cover a range of issues about the speed with which the service is delivered; a good example would be the use of POCT. The issues can then cover the impact of the use of POCT on the health outcome, which may cover impact on the clinical outcome and on cost. You will find it helpful to use "C" for "change" when looking at the evidence regarding operational changes.

Remember the range of operational outcome measures that were listed earlier in this book (Part 1).

Case 1. *The health maintenance organization (HMO) wants to investigate the costs and benefit of transferring more of the management of diabetes into the community setting. They also want to know if there is any evidence on the use of HbA1c testing in the ambulatory clinic or community care settings.*

Here is a situation in which setting is being considered, and so the use of the PICO variant to include "S" for "setting" is important.

P: patients with diabetes

I: POCT for HbA1c

C: laboratory testing for HbA1c

C: clinical decision on result at time of intervention

O: glycemic control

Question: Will the use of POCT for HbA1c as part of an integrated package of care for the management of diabetes improve glycemic control?

It is obvious that testing alone will not have any impact on outcomes. It is necessary to ensure that the result is used at the time of the clinic consultation as part of the disease management process.

❖❖❖

Case 2. *The chief executive of a large hospital is concerned that his emergency department is often unable to deal with patients immediately on admission and that waiting times are increasing. He asks the head of the laboratory if more rapid provision of test results would help to improve the triage of patients through the department.*

P: patients presenting to the emergency department

I: POCT

C: central laboratory testing

O: waiting times in the emergency department

Question: Will more rapid delivery of results in the emergency department using POCT reduce delays and improve triage times?*

* At this point the question is too broad and it will be necessary to identify which tests are likely to be of greatest value to the emergency medicine specialists.

❖❖❖

Case 3. *An HMO has received a proposal for coumadin (warfarin) monitoring in the community pharmacy to improve access for patients, to reduce the demand for hospital outpatient visits, and to improve health outcomes. The hematologist is asked to advise on the merit of the proposal.*

P: patients on coumadin therapy

I: INR testing in the community pharmacy

C: INR testing in the hospital ambulatory clinic

O: health outcomes, e.g., time spent in the therapeutic range

Is a PICO variant relevant here? Yes; there is change in setting—which in this case may be most associated with the change in the clinical environment. Are there adequate facilities available for the consultation?

Question: Does the management of patients on coumadin therapy by monitoring of the INR in the community pharmacy setting lead to improved patient outcomes and reduce demand for hospital clinic visits?**

** Clearly there are a number of questions that could be asked around this topic based on different outcomes.

❖❖❖

Now You Try It

Read the case below. Apply the PICO principle. Then develop a search question just as in the examples above. You can check your answers in the box below.

Case 4. *The head of the Women's and Children's Directorate has noticed that following the introduction of screening for* Chlamydia *using a PCR-based method, 25% of the patients screened do not return for the second consultation to receive the results (and hence treatment). She is aware that a POCT device for* Chlamydia *using the PCR method has recently become available. She wants to undertake a study to determine whether testing during the first visit leads to better health outcomes.*

P: ....

I: ....

C: ....

O: ....

In this situation it may be helpful to add "C" for "change" because a key part of this scenario is that the patient is treated at the time that the test result is produced.

Question:

....

....

❖❖❖

Possible Answers

P: women participating in a *Chlamydia* screening program

I: use of POCT for *Chlamydia*

C: use of central laboratory testing for *Chlamydia*

O: incidence of complications associated with *Chlamydia* infection

Question: Will the use of POCT for *Chlamydia* lead to a reduction in the complications associated with *Chlamydia* infection?

P: women participating in a *Chlamydia* screening program

I: use of POCT for *Chlamydia*

C: use of central laboratory testing for *Chlamydia*

O: number of clinic visits

Question: Will the use of POCT for *Chlamydia* lead to an impact on the number of clinic visits associated with the diagnosis and management of *Chlamydia* infection?

Your Own Cases

Choose two cases in your own institution that have come up in your laboratory practice. List them here. Then practice applying the PICO principle to these cases.

> Remember to think about PICO variants. If you choose to use one, or more, of them, then highlight with a note.

Case 5. ....

....

P: ....

I: ....

C: ....

(C): ....

O: ....

Question:

....

....

❖❖❖

Case 6. ....

....

P: ....

I: ....

C: ....

(C): ....

O: ....

Question:

....

....

❖❖❖

Economic

Health economic issues in the field of diagnostic testing are complex. However, they provide an opportunity to assess the cost of the test against the value or benefit that its use generates. Further, this assessment identifies where that benefit occurs and therefore where the gain will be realized.

It is likely that one, or more, of the PICO variants—perhaps "setting" and "change" (management) will be relevant to all of these cases. Economic considerations are invariably about a change in practice.

This knowledge helps to inform reconfiguration of the resource allocation as well as the change in the process of care that should occur to achieve the benefits claimed.

Case 1. *The public health physicians and health policymakers are concerned about the increasing prevalence of complications associated with* Chlamydia. *They wish to consider the health economic arguments in favor of a screening program in young women.*

P: young women aged 18 to 30 years old

I: screening for the presence of *Chlamydia* infection

C: no screening

O: costs of managing complications of *Chlamydia* infection

Question: Will the introduction of a screening program for *Chlamydia* in young women reduce the prevalence of complications associated with the infection?*

* It is obvious that testing alone will not have any impact on outcomes and that it is necessary to ensure that the result is used to inform treatment decisions.

❖❖❖

Case 2. *The chief executive of a large hospital is concerned that his emergency department is often unable to deal with patients immediately on admission and that waiting times are increasing. Evidence from a trial shows that POCT for four parameters generate a significant improvement in waiting and triage times. However, it is necessary to understand the costs associated with the use of POCT and where the benefits are seen elsewhere in the system, in order to inform resource allocation.*

P: patients being admitted to the emergency department

I: POCT

C: central laboratory testing

O: (i) additional costs of use of POCT, (ii) savings, and (iii) where these savings occur.

Question: Can the costs of rapid delivery of results in the emergency department using POCT be offset by reduction in costs elsewhere in the hospital, or by the generation of additional revenue?

❖❖❖

Case 3. *A clinical chemist wishes to introduce a test for BNP. His reasoning: it will enable rule-out of heart failure and thereby reduce the need for echocardiography in patients presenting to primary care with symptoms suggesting heart failure.*

P: patients presenting to primary care with symptoms suggestive of heart failure

I: BNP testing

C: no BNP testing

O: total cost of diagnosing heart failure

T: over a period of one year.*

* The choice of one year is based on the fact: the evidence shows that BNP testing can reduce the need for echocardiography in all patients, and so the reduced cost will come from performing fewer "echo's" as well as reduced clinic time.

Question: Does the introduction of BNP as a first-line test in the diagnostic triage pathway for patients with suspected heart failure attending their primary care physician reduce the total cost involved in making the diagnosis of heart failure?

❖❖❖

Now You Try It

Read the case below. Apply the PICO principle. Then develop a search question just as in the examples above. You can check your answers in the box below.

Case 4. *After the introduction of screening for* Chlamydia *using a PCR-based method, the head of the Women's and Children's Directorate noticed that 25% of the patients screened do not return for the second consultation to receive the results. She is aware that a POCT device for* Chlamydia *using the PCR method has recently become available, and that early indications are that POCT ensures that the cost of follow up is reduced and more patients are treated. She wants to undertake a study to ascertain whether testing at the time of the first visit saves money.*

P: ....

I: ....

C: ....

O: ....

Question:

....

....

> Did you use any of the PICO variants in the cases above? If you chose to use one, or more, of them, then highlight with a note.

❖❖❖

Possible Answers

P: women participating in a *Chlamydia* screening program

I: use of POCT for *Chlamydia*

C: use of central laboratory testing for *Chlamydia*

O: number of cases referred with ectopic pregnancy, infertility, and/or pelvic inflammatory disease due to *Chlamydia* infection

Question: Will the use of POCT for *Chlamydia* lead to a reduction in the incidence of patients referred to the hospital with ectopic pregnancy, infertility, and/or pelvic inflammatory disease associated with *Chlamydia* infection?

The more direct question is this:

P: women participating in a *Chlamydia* screening program

I: use of POCT for *Chlamydia*

C: use of central laboratory testing for *Chlamydia*

O: cost of cases referred with ectopic pregnancy, infertility, and/or pelvic inflammatory disease due to *Chlamydia* infection

Question: Will the use of POCT for *Chlamydia* lead to a reduction in the hospital costs associated with patients referred to the hospital with ectopic pregnancy, infertility, and/or pelvic inflammatory disease associated with *Chlamydia* infection?

Your Own Cases

Choose two cases in your own institution that have come up in your laboratory practice. List them here. Then practice applying the PICO principle to these cases.

Remember to think about the PICO variants. If you choose to use one, or more, of them, then highlight with a note.

Case 5. ....

....

P: ....

I: ....

C: ....

O: ....

Question:

....

....

❖❖❖

Case 6. ....

....

P: ....

I: ....

C: ....

O: ....

Question:

....

....

❖❖❖

Taking Stock

So, what have you learned?

As a result of working through this section, you should now understand...

- That it's important to differentiate types of questions, e.g., foreground and background questions, as to their usefulness in helping solve a clinical problem
- How well-structured questions help clearly articulate the clinical problem requiring a solution
- That well-structured questions can be formulated guided by the **PICO** approach: i.e., considering **P**atient, **I**ntervention, **C**omparator, and **O**utcome
- How derivatives of PICO (prior test, setting, time, and change [management]) can assist in formulating well-structured questions
- How to apply the PICO approach to different settings, and including different perspectives

Some thoughts on how to get additional help if you still have concerns:

(i) talk to a colleague and try to resolve through discussion

(ii) talk it through with your tutor or mentor

(iii) post a question on a professional listserver or mailbase (e.g., the mailbase of the Association for Clinical Biochemistry in the United Kingdom [www.acb.org.uk])

(iv) find an EBLM expert and ask him/her (try professional associations, such as AACC [www.aacc.org] and the Centre for Evidence-Based Medicine [www.cebm.net])

Pause and Reflect

On a scale of 1 (poor) to 10 (excellent), now rate your skill in

(i) Identifying the elements of PICO ....

(ii) Differentiating the different types of questions ....

(iii) Applying PICO (and its derivatives) in different situations

Etiology ....

Screening ....

Diagnosis ....

Prognosis ....

Treatment ....

(iv) and from different perspectives

Analytical ....

Operational ....

Economic ....

(v) Applying PICO and its derivatives to your own case studies ....

Now look back at the concerns that you had before you started to go through the case studies (see page 52) and see if you still have those concerns.

....

....

....

....

Putting PICO into Practice

This process is an excellent practice to share with colleagues. (It's also an excellent resource for mentoring less experienced colleagues.) Why not make it the basis of a journal club?

References

1. Del Mar C, Doust J, Glasziou P. Clinical Thinking. Evidence, Communication and Decision-Making. Oxford: Blackwell Publishing BMJ Books, 2006:127pp.
2. Richardson WS, Wilson MC, Nishikawa J, Hayward RSA. The well built clinical question: a key to evidence-based decisions. AJP Journal 1995;123:A12–3.
3. Jackson R, Ameratunga S, Broad J. The GATE frame: critical appraisal with pictures. ACP J Club 2006;144:A8–11.

STEP A2: ACQUIRE—Find the Evidence

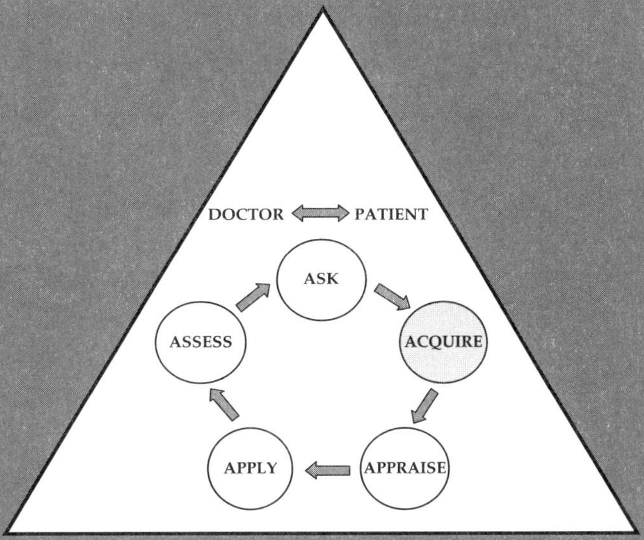

In this chapter

- Determining availability of evidence
- Insight into matching study design and types of questions
- Types of research and the use of primary vs. secondary literature
- Linking question and search strategy
- Where and how to search for evidence
- A sample search: steps in the process
- Applying PubMed features to a research question

Acquire: Searching for (and Finding) the Evidence

Once the topic of interest is formulated into an answerable question using the PICO strategy, you can begin the process of ACQUIRING the evidence.

The first approach to answering the question is to evaluate if there is any evidence that addresses the issue. If there is a significant body of evidence, then you might consider a systematic review of the literature. Typically you take this approach when seeking definitive statements on the use of a test: for example, when considering the development of a guideline or care pathway. This process can be illustrated as a flow diagram (see figure in sidebar).

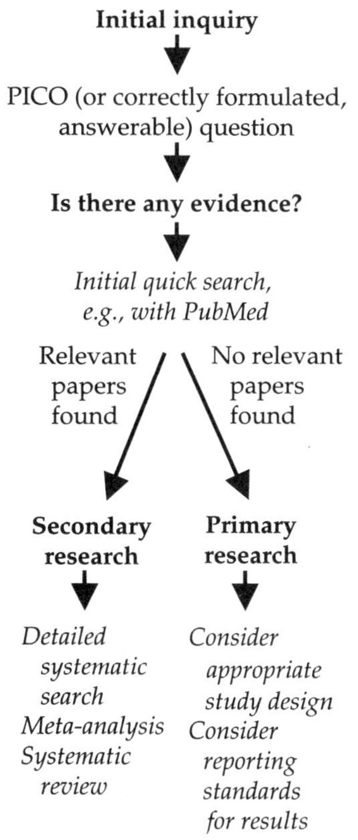

If there is a paucity of evidence, the formulated question may be the basis for a research project. Here, the question aids in guiding the enrollment criteria, clinical setting, comparator, outcome measures, and appropriate study design.

Appropriate study design is critical for minimizing bias in answering the question. The table on page 92 summarizes some of the issues and characteristics involved in appropriate study design and can be used to both narrow the universe of articles for systematic review (in the case of abundant relevant evidence) and to guide study design (in the case of no relevant evidence). Though designing a research project is beyond the scope of this workbook, detailed information on study design is provided in Appendix A.

Key Concept

A significant body of evidence indicates that undertaking a systematic review of the evidence to answer the research question may be productive. A paucity of evidence calls for designing a research project in a way that provides best evidence and minimizes bias.

Types of Questions and Associated Study Design*

Type of question	Type of follow-up	Recommended design	Comment
Diagnostic accuracy	Cross-sectional	Cohort study	Should be a consecutive group of patients. Should be blind comparison between the index test and the reference method (gold standard).
Therapy or prevention	Longitudinal	Randomized controlled trial (RCT)	Subjects randomly allocated to treatment or control arms.
Impact on decision-making (test/no test)	Longitudinal	RCT	Assessing impact of having the test available vs. no test available.
Prognosis	Longitudinal	Cohort study	Association of test results with outcomes for relevant cohort.
Risk factors or exploratory analysis	Longitudinal ("follow-back")	Case-control	Subjects with outcome (cases) and without (controls) matched and compared for initial risk factors, results of new markers, etc.

*A detailed explanation of each type of study can be found in Appendix A.

Types of Research

Primary research refers to the performance of individual studies. These can be randomized controlled trials (RCTs), various types of cohort studies, case-control design, etc. (see table on page 92).

Secondary research is an endeavor that reviews and, when appropriate, combines and summarizes information from primary research to gain insights from the cumulative experience of the studies in the specific topic area. The collective information from secondary research is valuable. You can specify searches for secondary research articles when using electronic databases (as will be discussed later).

Systematic review is a most important type of secondary research in which evidence (from primary studies) that addresses a specifically formulated question is systematically identified, appraised, and combined with the goal of obtaining a summary and a reliable overview of the dependable evidence. Systematic reviews begin with a structured clinical question and a thorough search of the literature (see next section). None of the individual primary studies may be able to answer the question fully; however, the reviewers seek to combine the identified evidence and, when appropriate, collate and pool the information. A measure of reason (or caution) is typically necessary after locating primary evidence to evaluate if it is consistent and "makes sense." (When it is not consistent, i.e., when there is extreme variation in primary data, it is described as having "heterogeneity.") There may be methodological and/or clinical reasons why pooling of data does not make sense, such as when the primary results are conflicting. In these cases, investigators typically use summary tables that display the data in a transparent way such that the methods, clinical characteristics of populations, and results from the primary studies can be easily examined by readers. When data are relatively homogeneous, a meta-analysis may be appropriate.

Meta-analysis is a formal statistical procedure that combines results of primary studies in an effort to provide the best overall estimate of the average common effect and confidence interval (CI). Meta-analysis is conducted whenever possible and included in systematic reviews because they can assist in minimizing sampling variation, they can help provide useful insights when single studies are underpowered, and they can estimate more precisely the test performance, treatment effect, etc. Meta-analysis results are typically displayed as Forest plots that show the results of individual primary studies, for example, the use of turbidimetric D-dimer testing in the diagnosis of pulmonary embolism *(1)*. Typically, filled circles represent the mean effect size of each study and the horizontal lines represent the 95% CI [see figure in sidebar for use of D-dimer in diagnosing pulmonary embolism *(1)*].

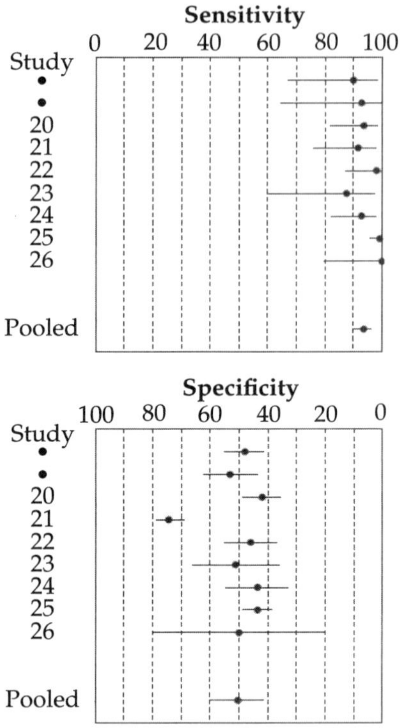

Key Concept

Secondary research sources of evidence are preferred for addressing most questions because experts have extracted, rated, and reviewed the information. Primary studies are also valuable, particularly when they more specifically address the questions and include the populations of interest. When searching for evidence, take care to assure that the type of question matches the study design (refer to table on page 92).

How to Search for, and Acquire, Evidence

Twenty years ago the conventional advice about retrieving information would have involved trudging to your institution's library to conduct a hand search using hard copy periodicals. Today, however, the only realistic option for searching is to utilize the power of the internet.

The Clinical Question Drives the Search

The search strategy should be directed by elements in the formulated question (refer to table on page 92) and use of Boolean logic terms (see figure in sidebar and table on page 100).

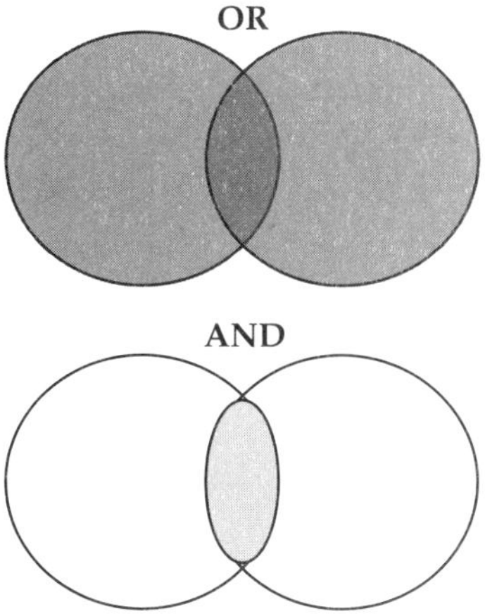

Boolean search operators

The search itself may utilize a number of internet resources (see table below and Part 3 of this workbook). Of these, PubMed must be considered the most useful source for searching in everyday practice, e.g., when receiving a telephone call, a visit from a clinician, or on ward rounds. (Such ad hoc searches are often referred to as "quick and dirty.") PubMed has a rich archive of literature, is well maintained with frequent updates, and is readily accessible at no cost.

Consulting a professional trained in library science is the most effective way of conducting a search, particularly when one needs to be truly comprehensive. In this case it is also useful to have a multidisciplinary team that can help to formulate the questions, help identify search terms, and evaluate the output of the searching process *(2, 3)*. These comprehensive searches are covered elsewhere (see Reference 2) and are beyond the scope of what will be covered here.

Databases and Descriptions That May Be Useful for Locating Evidence

MEDLINE (PubMed)
http://www.pubmed.gov
The most popular and widely used resource for quick searches. Contains more than 10 million citations going back to the mid-1960s. PubMed is free and is produced by the U.S. National Library of Medicine.

Web of Science
http://scientific.thomson.com/products/wos/
Provides a multi-disciplinary approach to accessing current and previous information from about 8,700 high-impact journals. Users can navigate to the full-text version of journal articles.

Continued

Databases and Descriptions That May Be Useful for Locating Evidence (Cont'd)

The Cochrane Library
http://www.Cochrane.org
Contains several databases, including The Cochrane Database of Systematic Reviews, The Database of Abstracts of Reviews of Effects (DARE), and the Cochrane Central Register of Controlled Trials (CENTRAL). Although this is an extensive resource, most of the information concerns therapeutic and interventional trials and very little laboratory medicine.

ACP Journal Club
http://hiru.mcmaster.ca/acpjc/default.htm
Selects original studies and systematic reviews from the biomedical literature that merit immediate attention by physicians attempting to keep pace with important advances in internal medicine. These articles are summarized in abstracts with commentary by clinical experts.

TRIP (Turning Research into Practice)
http://www.tripdatabase.com/aboutus/index.html
Facile means of answering clinical questions using evidence-based medicine techniques. Medical images are included as well as patient information leaflets. A search box is utilized for input of information.

MEDION
http://www.mediondatabase.nl
Produced by investigators at the universities of Maastricht (the Netherlands) and Leuven (Belgium) with a special interest in diagnostic studies and diagnostic reviews. Includes the references and abstracts of published studies.

EMBASE
http://www.embase.com
Proprietary database that contains a number of citations not found within MEDLINE.

Exercise: Walking through a Sample Search

1. **Use PICO to formulate the question and the search terms**. The PICO format is again convenient to use for deriving the search terms; the search may be structured by specifying:

   [**P**opulation OR synonym(s)] AND

   [**I**ntervention OR synonym(s)] AND

   [**C**omparator OR synonym(s)] AND

   [**O**utcome OR synonym(s)]

> Remember the PICO variants. For example, you may wish to consider "S" for setting;" in any case, you should ensure that if the setting might be relevant that it is covered in the "P" component.

Here's an example:

Question: *In adults arriving at the emergency department with signs and symptoms of acute coronary syndrome, does a natriuretic peptide measurement help to predict risk of 1-year mortality?*

Question part	Interpretation of term	Synonym
Population	Adult, emergency department Acute coronary syndrome	Heart attack, unstable angina, myocardial ischemia
Intervention	Elevated B-type natriuretic peptide (BNP)	Elevated NT-proBNP
Comparator	None, patients with low BNP values	None, lower NT-proBNP values
Outcome	1-year mortality	Death at 12 months

2. **Broadly identify the type of question.** In this case, it is prognostic (Note: In the case of a cohort study, there may not be a control group, i.e., "C"of PICO).
3. **Identify the type of search.** We will conduct a detailed systematic search, seeking out cohort studies because their longitudinal follow-up is useful for predicting outcomes.
4. **Choose the appropriate database.** We will use MEDLINE (www.pubmed.gov).
5. **Identify keywords and MeSH terms.** Terms that are central to the question and the resulting search are called "keywords." In the example above, you might first locate articles that include the keyword natriuretic peptide (BNP or NT-proBNP) in relation to patients with acute coronary syndrome. However you might wonder if the synonyms identified the most appropriate terms for the topic. The "Medical Subject Headings" (MeSH) feature of PubMed can help address this issue.

   MeSH terms comprise a controlled vocabulary, also called descriptors, that describe the content of articles in the PubMed database. These descriptors are as specific as possible to help focus the search and demonstrate the hierarchy of terms used by the PubMed database. In other words, MeSH terms indicate the topic of an article, rather than a keyword that simply retrieves the paper if the word or term appears. You can also use MeSH to

Overview: Steps in the Search Process

1. Use PICO to formulate the question (and to derive search terms).
2. Broadly identify type of question (diagnostic, therapy or prevention, prognostic, etc.).
3. Identify the type of search (detailed systematic search, systematic review, meta-analysis, etc.) most likely to yield the best evidence for the type of question being asked.
4. Choose the appropriate database (PubMed is most useful for everyday practice; see table on pages 95 and 96 for additional databases).
5. Identify keywords and MeSH terms; perform search.
6. Narrow search terms as needed, and apply relevant Boolean commands (see table on page 100).
7. Retrieve types of studies relevant to type of question (step 2, above; see also table on page 92).
8. Save relevant articles to PubMed clipboard for review and appraisal.

help identify additional terms that may be appropriate for a search. In the example, using the MeSH option in PubMed and entering "acute coronary syndrome" retrieves the following hierarchy:

Entry Terms:

- Acute Coronary Syndromes
- Coronary Syndrome, Acute
- Coronary Syndromes, Acute
- Syndrome, Acute Coronary
- Syndromes, Acute Coronary

All MeSH Categories
- Diseases Category
  - Cardiovascular Diseases
    - Heart Diseases
      - Myocardial Ischemia
        - **Acute Coronary Syndrome**

Thus "Acute Coronary Syndrome" is a subset under "Myocardial Ischemia" in PubMed. Selecting "Myocardial Ischemia" displays numerous other relevant terms.

Myocardial Ischemia
- Acute Coronary Syndrome
- Angina Pectoris
  - Angina, Unstable +
  - Microvascular Angina
- Coronary Disease
  - Coronary Aneurysm
  - Coronary Artery Disease
  - Coronary Occlusion
  - Coronary Stenosis +
  - Coronary Thrombosis
  - Coronary Vasospasm
- Myocardial Infarction
  - Myocardial Stunning
  - No-Reflow Phenomenon
  - Shock, Cardiogenic
- Myocardial Reperfusion Injury
- Myocardial Stunning

6. **Narrow search terms as needed, and apply relevant Boolean commands** (see table on page 100). If the term "Myocardial Ischemia" is too broad for your question, the PubMed MeSH feature provides other search terms that may help you retrieve relevant articles.

   After examining the MeSH terms, you may decide that "Myocardial Ischemia" is a better term to use to form the Boolean combination between the population (myocardial ischemia), the intervention or test (BNP), and the outcome (mortality) in the formulated question. (See figure in sidebar.)

   When searching, a productive strategy is to systematically step through the process. We can start this search with this statement:

   (BNP OR NT-proBNP) AND (Myocardial Ischemia)

   Articles that examine the relationship between a natriuretic peptide and an outcome of mortality can be retrieved this way:

   (BNP OR NT-proBNP) AND (Mortality)

   These Boolean relationships form the basis of searching for articles that may be relevant to your question. Many complex relationships between, and among, the elements of the formulated question can be derived. In addition to the "AND" and "OR" Boolean operators that are commonly used in searching, there are a number of other commands that are useful depending on the circumstances (see table on page 100).

7. **Retrieve types of studies relevant to type of question.** Because the question is prognostic, we have decided to retrieve as many cohort studies as possible.

8. **Save relevant articles to clipboard for review and appraisal.** PubMed allows you to select the studies you want to review and save them to a clipboard for downloading or printing. This speeds the retrieval process, making it less tedious and ultimately more efficient and effective.

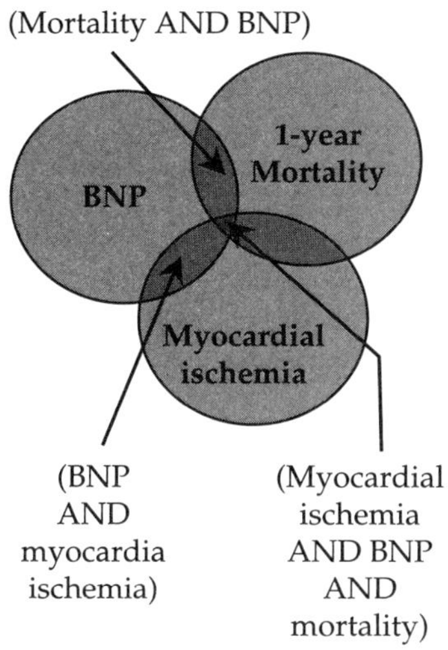

Selected PubMed Boolean Commands

Command	Description
OR	Retrieves articles containing either word or phrase. For example, searching on *Alanine transaminase OR Aspartate transaminase* will retrieve articles with either *Alanine transaminase* or *Aspartate transaminase.*
AND	Retrieves articles containing both words or phrases. For example, searching on *Alanine transaminase AND Aspartate transaminase* will only retrieve articles that contain both phrases.
NOT	Retrieves articles containing one word or phrase but not articles with the other. For example, searching on *Alanine transaminase NOT Aspartate transaminase* will retrieve articles containing *Alanine transaminase* and exclude those containing *Aspartate transaminase.*
Limits	This is a strategy to retrieve articles limited by date, language, those containing an abstract, and so on.
Parenthesis ( )	This can be used to group words or phrases, for example, (*Alanine transaminase OR Aspartate transaminase*) AND (*Hepatitis B OR Cholestasis*).
Asterisk *	This is a "wild card" that can be used in truncating words and instructing the search engine to retrieve the word stem and any variations of the word. For example, searching on *Hepat** will retrieve words with the *hepat* stem, such as *Hepatitis*, *Hepatoma*, etc.
[ti]	Retrieves words in the title. For example, searching on *Hepatitis [ti]* will only find studies with the term *Hepatitis* in the title.
MeSH	U.S. National Library of Medicine's controlled vocabulary; it is used for indexing articles for MEDLINE/PubMed. MeSH terminology provides a consistent way to retrieve information that may use different terminology for the same concepts. The vocabulary of keywords may also be used in PubMed or the Cochrane collection.

Applying PubMed's Special Features to a Research Question

Let's walk through another example, this time using special features such as "Clinical Queries," "Limits," etc.

Internet access is ubiquitous, so it will be assumed that navigating to the MEDLINE internet site at http://www.ncbi.nlm.nih.gov/sites/entrez/ (or simply, www.pubmed.gov) and finding the PubMed page below is straightforward. To conduct a search, you can enter keywords and the Boolean strategy into the search box circled at the upper portion of the search page. Note the "MeSH Database" feature (discussed earlier) and the "Clinical Queries" options (PubMed screen shot 1), which are highlighted on the left side of the main screen. The "Clinical Queries" option allows a researcher to select the clinical category of interest (etiology, diagnosis, etc.) and the search's scope, i.e., "broad" vs. "narrow" (PubMed screen shot 2.) Note that it is necessary to input your searching strategy into the "Clinical Queries" search box rather than the main entry term box.

Other useful features of PubMed include the "Limits" tab (PubMed screen shot 3). This feature allows the searcher to specify languages, types of articles, and subsets of topics as well as ages of the population (PubMed screen shot 4).

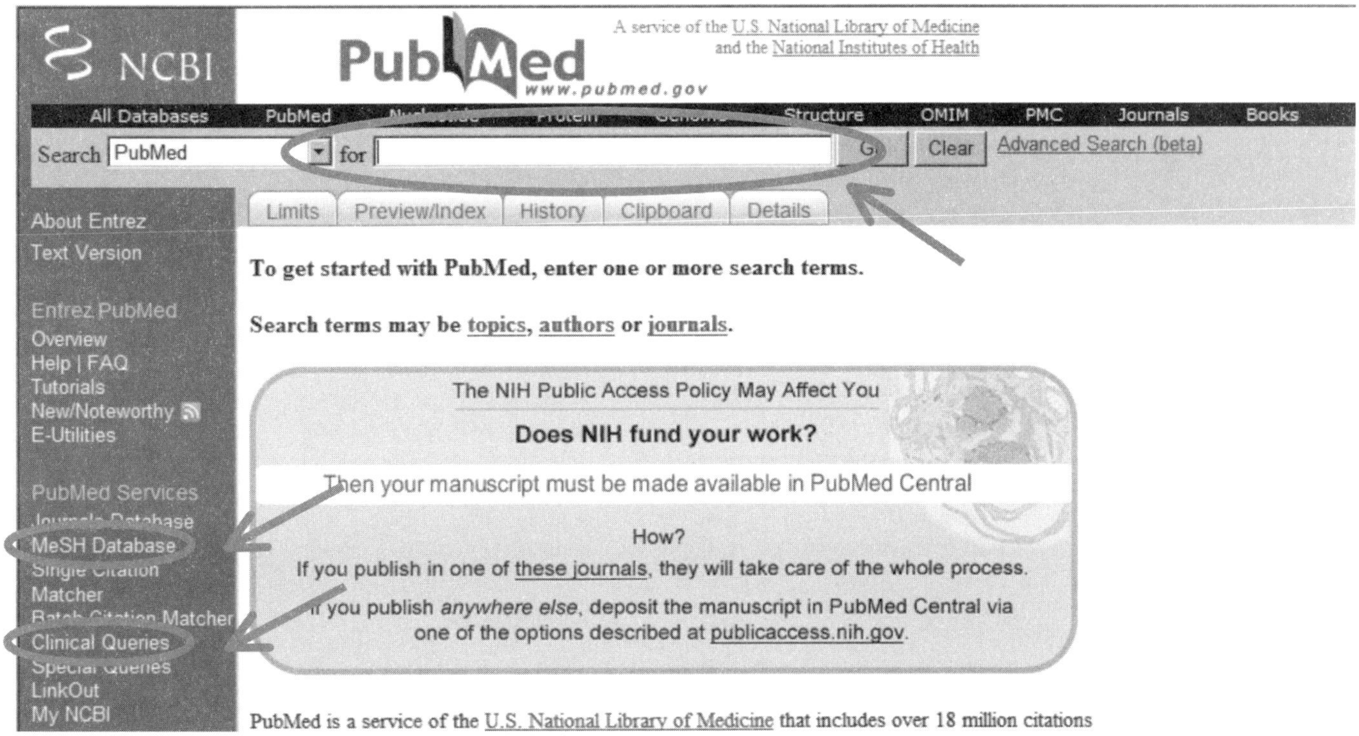

PubMed screen shot 1

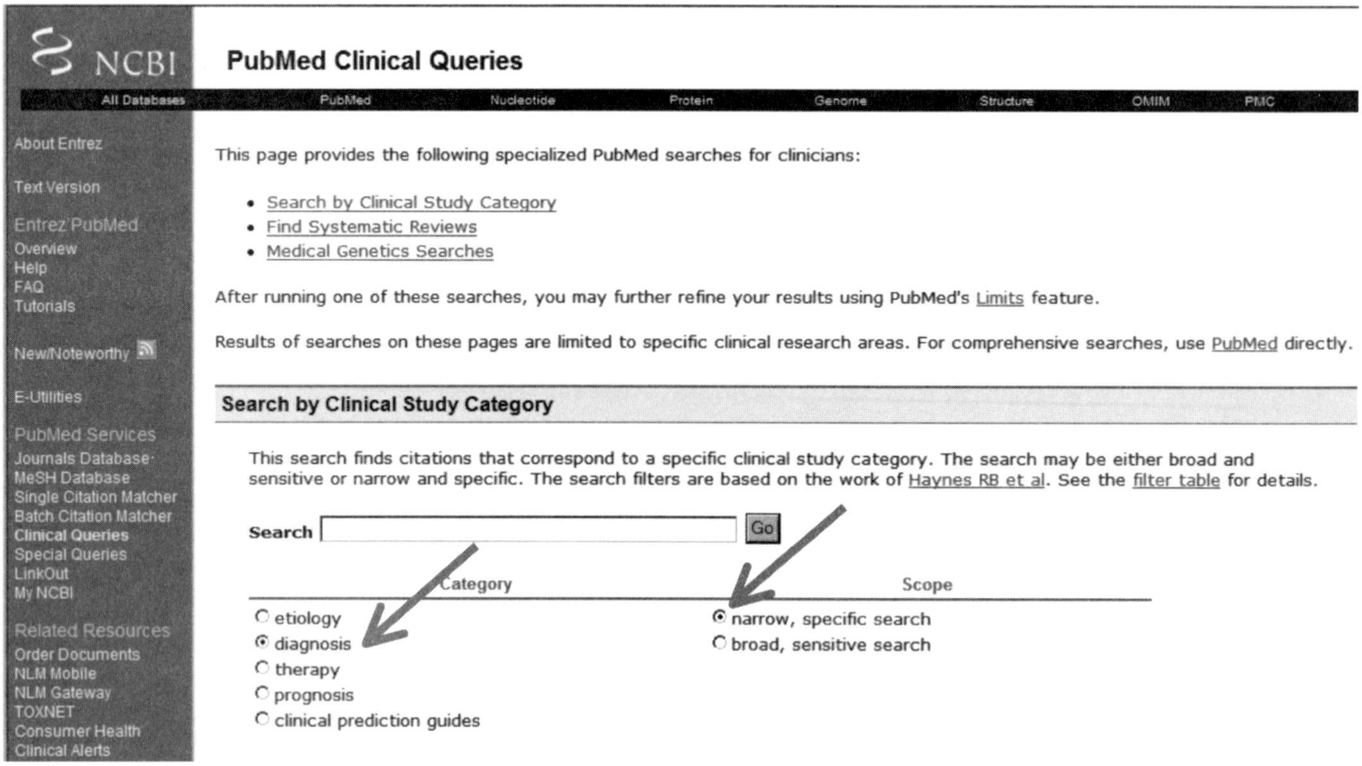

PubMed screen shot 2

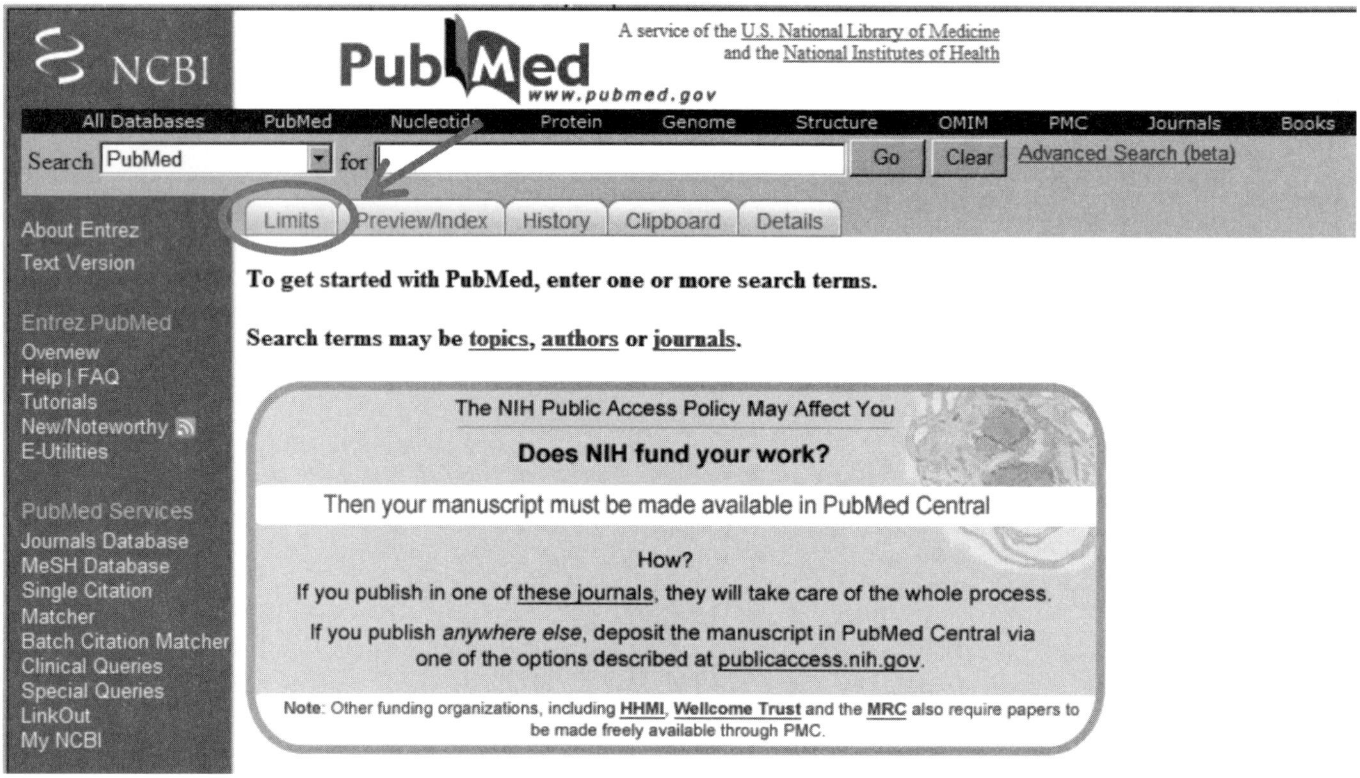

PubMed screen shot 3

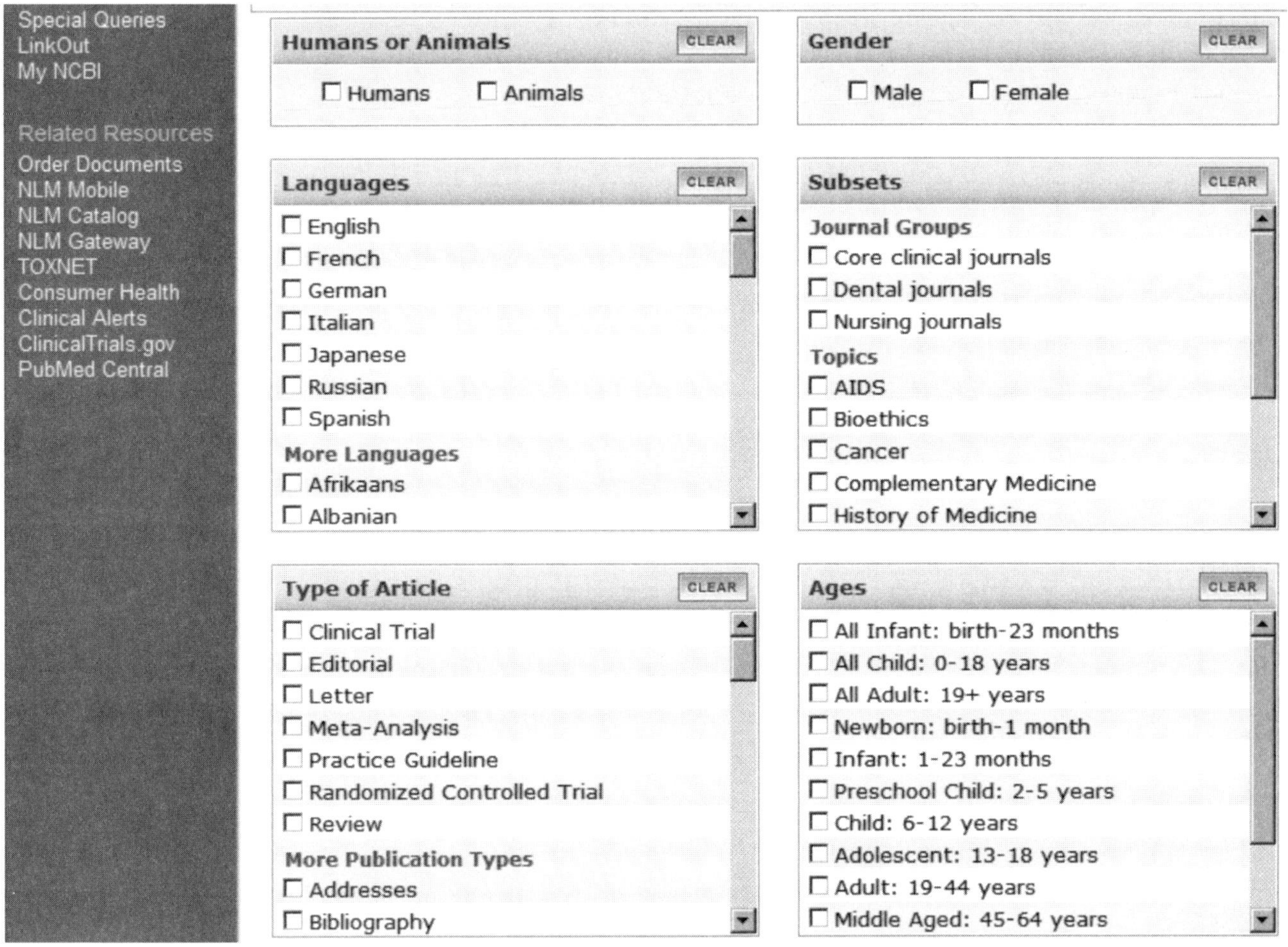

PubMed screen shot 4

The following example illustrates how to use these features in finding relevant evidence.

Case. *Your emergency department chair has approached you about offering D-dimer testing as an aid for the diagnosis of pulmonary embolism in symptomatic patients presenting to their service. There is an emergency medicine faculty meeting in two days in which he would like you to present your impressions on this testing.*

Applying PICO yields the following question:

What is the performance of D-Dimer for diagnosis of pulmonary embolism in patients presenting to the emergency department?

You underline terms that will be important for your search:

What is the performance of ***D-Dimer*** *for* ***diagnosis*** *of* ***pulmonary embolism*** *in patients presenting to the* ***emergency department****?*

> Note that the setting is specifically identified in the search.

Using the MeSH database and entering "pulmonary embolism," you find the following hierarchy:

- Cardiovascular Diseases
  - Vascular Diseases
    - Embolism and Thrombosis
      - Embolism
        - **Pulmonary Embolism**
          - Pulmonary Infarction

The emergency medicine chair asked specifically about "pulmonary embolism" so you decide to use this term, realizing that "pulmonary infarction" articles will also be retrieved. You access PubMed, enter the search [pulmonary embolism AND D-dimer], and receive your response (PubMed screen shot 5).

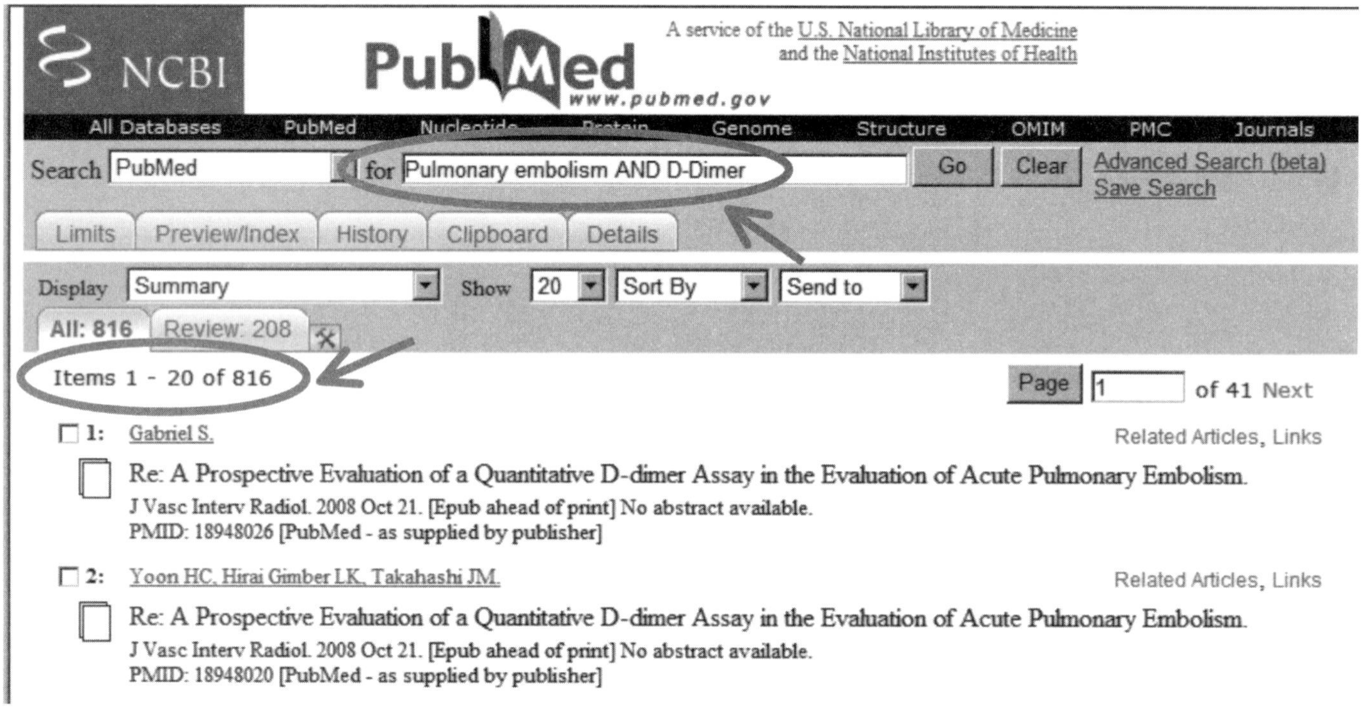

PubMed screen shot 5

There are 816 citations that include some aspect of this relationship! The search must be limited, so you choose the "Limits" tab, and select papers in English. Also, time is short so you examine the secondary research evidence available; you check the "Meta-Analysis" (or "systematic review") and the "Practice Guideline" boxes shown in the center screen (PubMed screen shot 6).

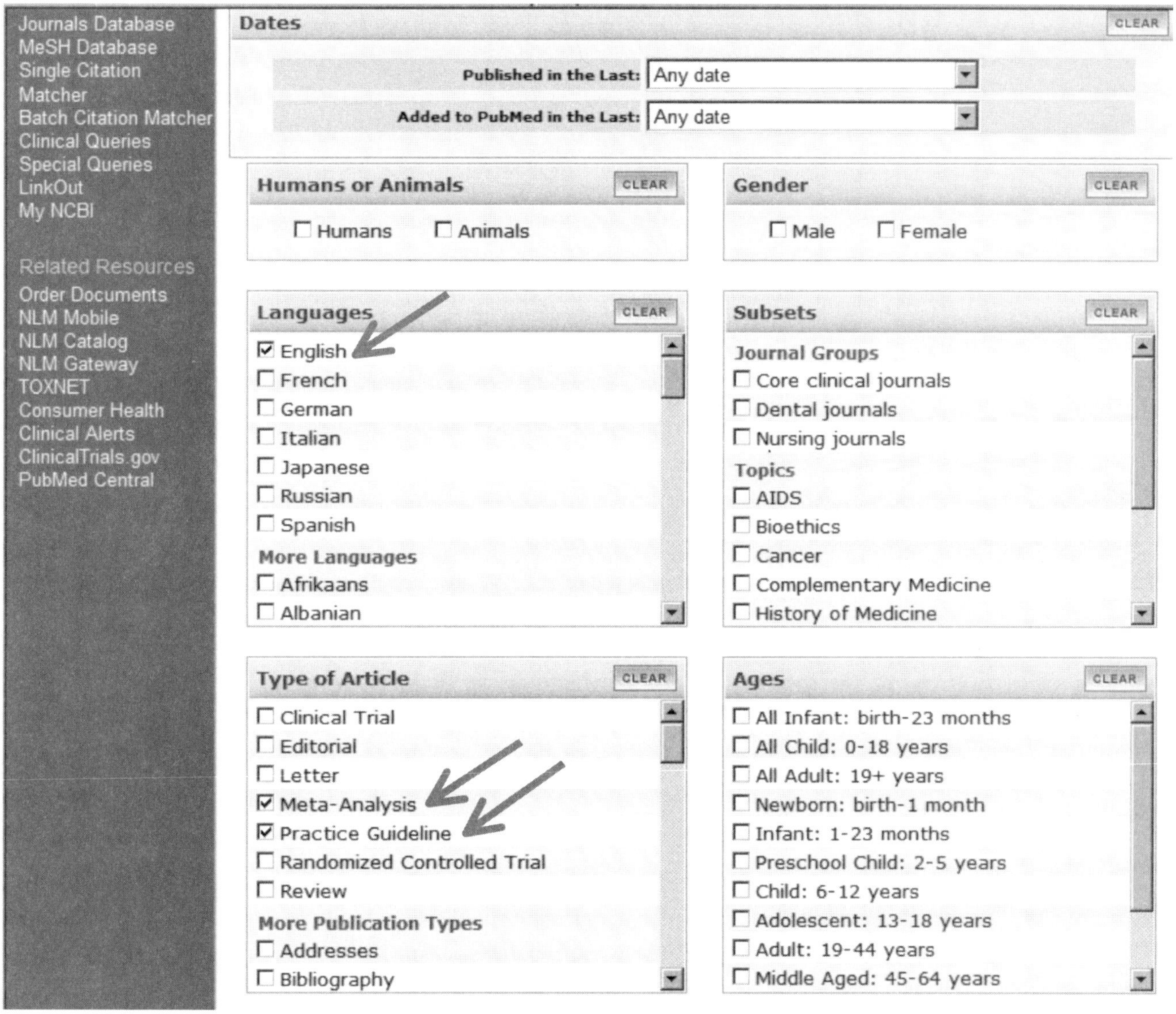

PubMed screen shot 6

The screen shows 16 articles that are literature summaries in English (PubMed screen shot 7).

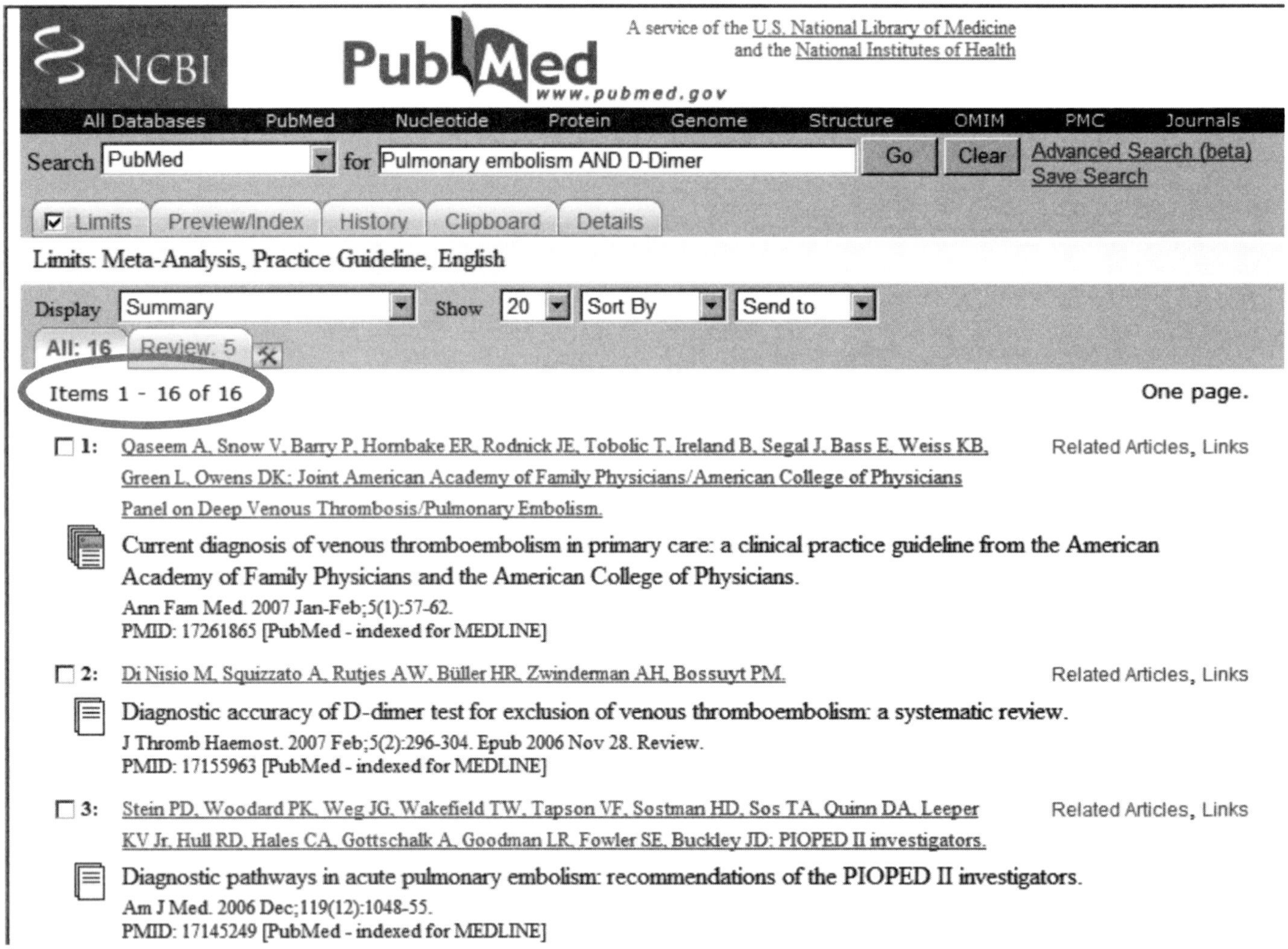

PubMed screen shot 7

Sixteen is a reasonably manageable number; however, you wish to see if the search can be narrowed further. To do this you choose the "Clinical Queries" option and make the selections shown (PubMed screen shot 8). This further restricts the number of articles to five (PubMed screen shot 9).

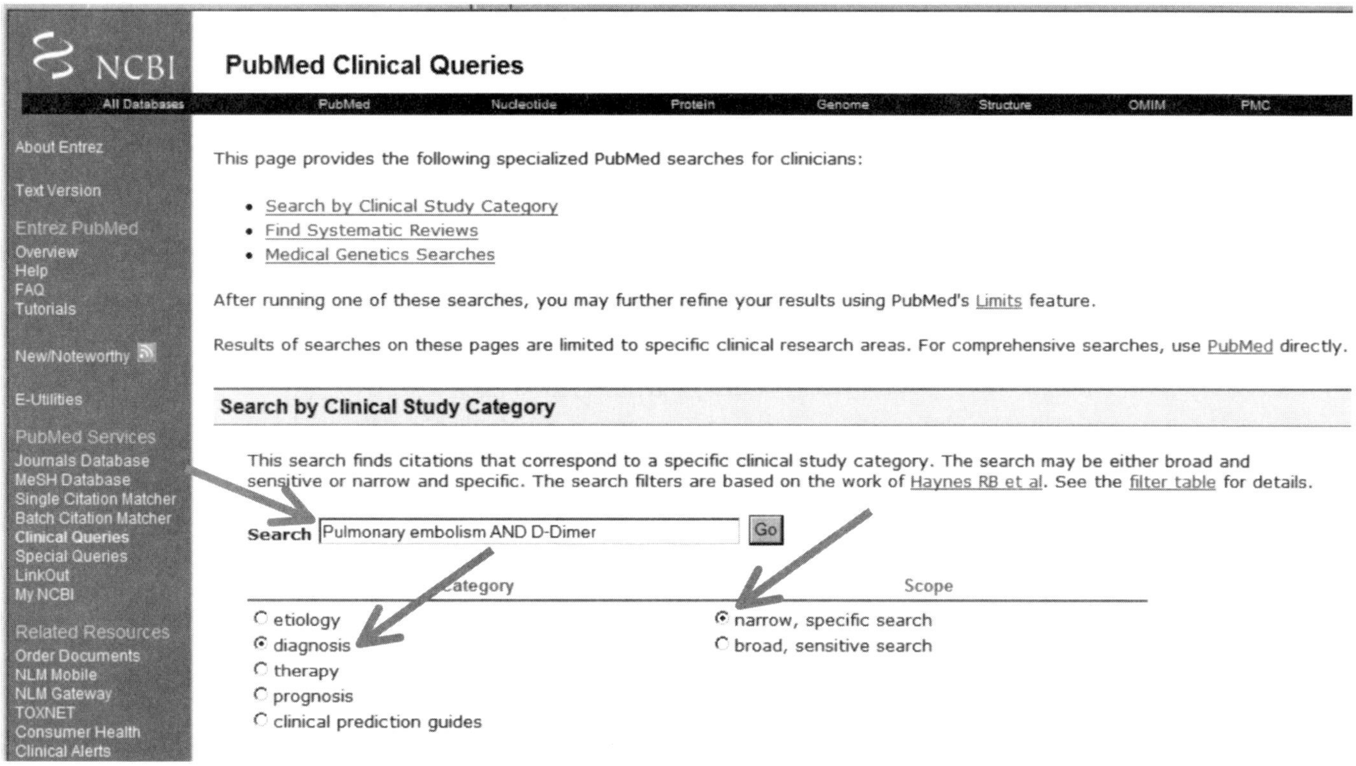

PubMed screen shot 8

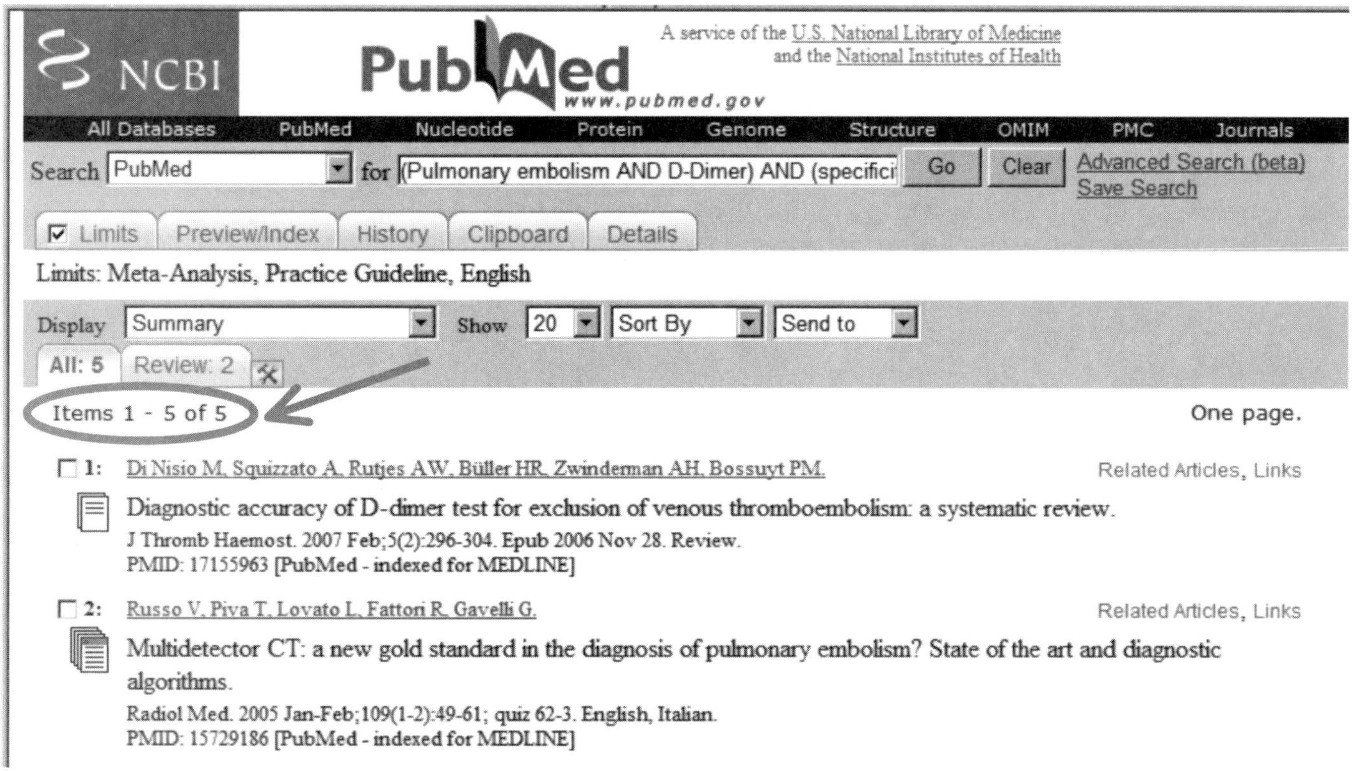

PubMed screen shot 9

Try this:

Duplicate the steps of the search above on your own computer. What number of articles would have been retrieved if you had selected "broad" rather than "narrow" in the "Clinical Queries" feature of PubMed for the search above?

Note: "Broad" and "narrow" searching is a convenience because the Boolean search is entered automatically for you. In this case, the difference between the "narrow" and "broad" search strategies is as follows:

Narrow

(pulmonary embolism AND d-dimer) AND
(specificity[Title/Abstract])

Broad

(pulmonary embolism AND d-dimer) AND
(sensitiv*[Title/Abstract] OR
sensitivity and specificity[MeSH Terms] OR
diagnos*[Title/Abstract] OR
diagnosis[MeSH:noexp] OR
diagnostic *[MeSH:noexp] OR
diagnosis,differential[MeSH:noexp] OR
diagnosis[Subheading:noexp])

Use of the "Narrow" search simply includes the Boolean intersection of your search terms with "specificity" in the title and abstract. The "broad" search is obviously much more involved, including both sensitivity and specificity, along with various wild cards and MeSH terms. Therefore using these "Clinical Queries" features has facilitated your task by doing much of the work of designing searches for you.

Key Concept

You can make your searches more manageable by specifying selections in PubMed's special features ("Clinical Queries," "Limits," "Search Scope," etc.). Using the "broad" vs. "narrow" options will also create an "automatic" Boolean search string.

When One Thing Leads to Another

The process of acquiring evidence frequently leads to other questions. An example might be the following.

You are aware that pulmonary embolism's associated condition, deep vein thrombosis (or venous thromboembolism), can also be of concern to emergency medicine physicians. So you wonder about the diagnostic performance of D-dimer in venous thromboembolism. You decide to search again, using the same limits as you did earlier, and the "Clinical Queries" feature (PubMed screen shot 10).

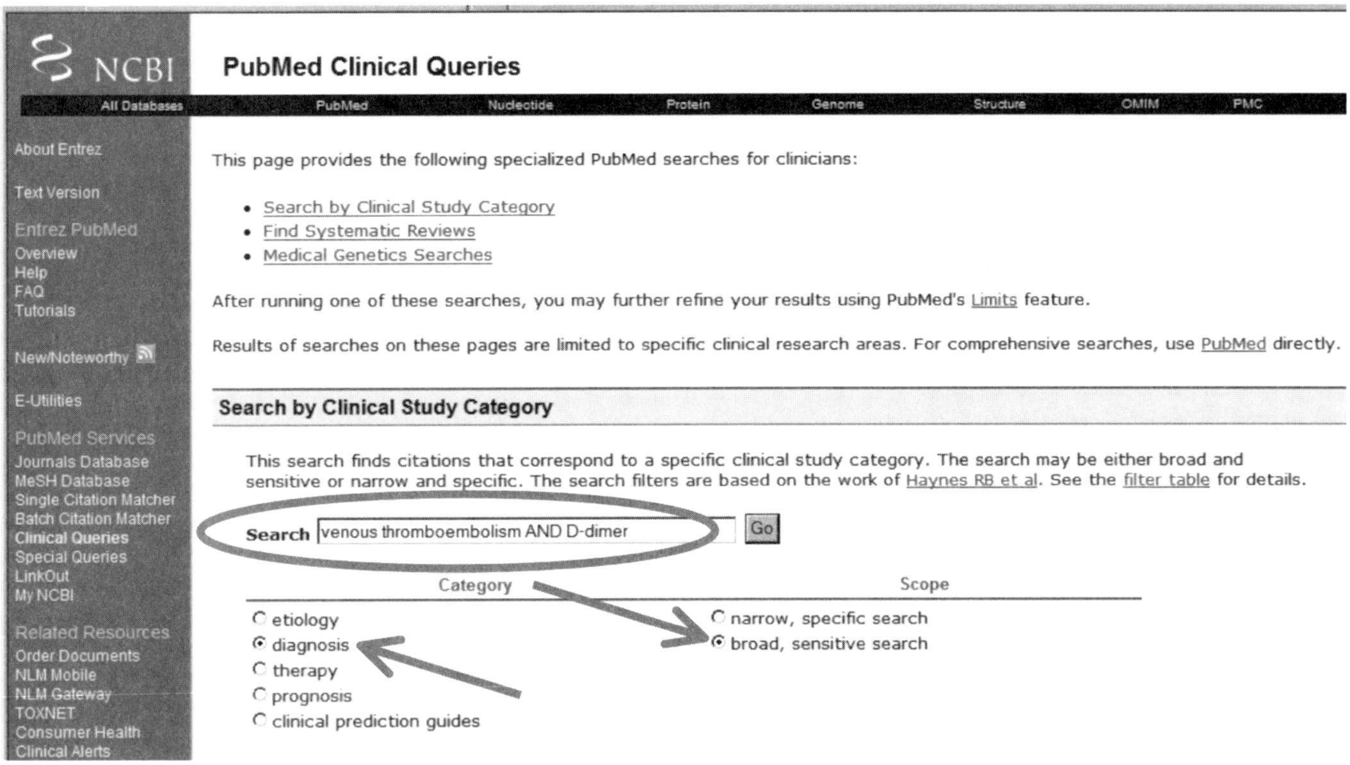

PubMed screen shot 10

Even with a broad search only two papers are retrieved (PubMed screen shot 11). Note that you can see the full text of each article that is available without cost.

Unfortunately the full text of all literature is not accessible without cost from PubMed due to restrictions by some publishers. However, institutional libraries often have paid subscriptions that allow access. Alternatively, a PDF of the paper can often be obtained by emailing the primary or corresponding author listed for the paper.

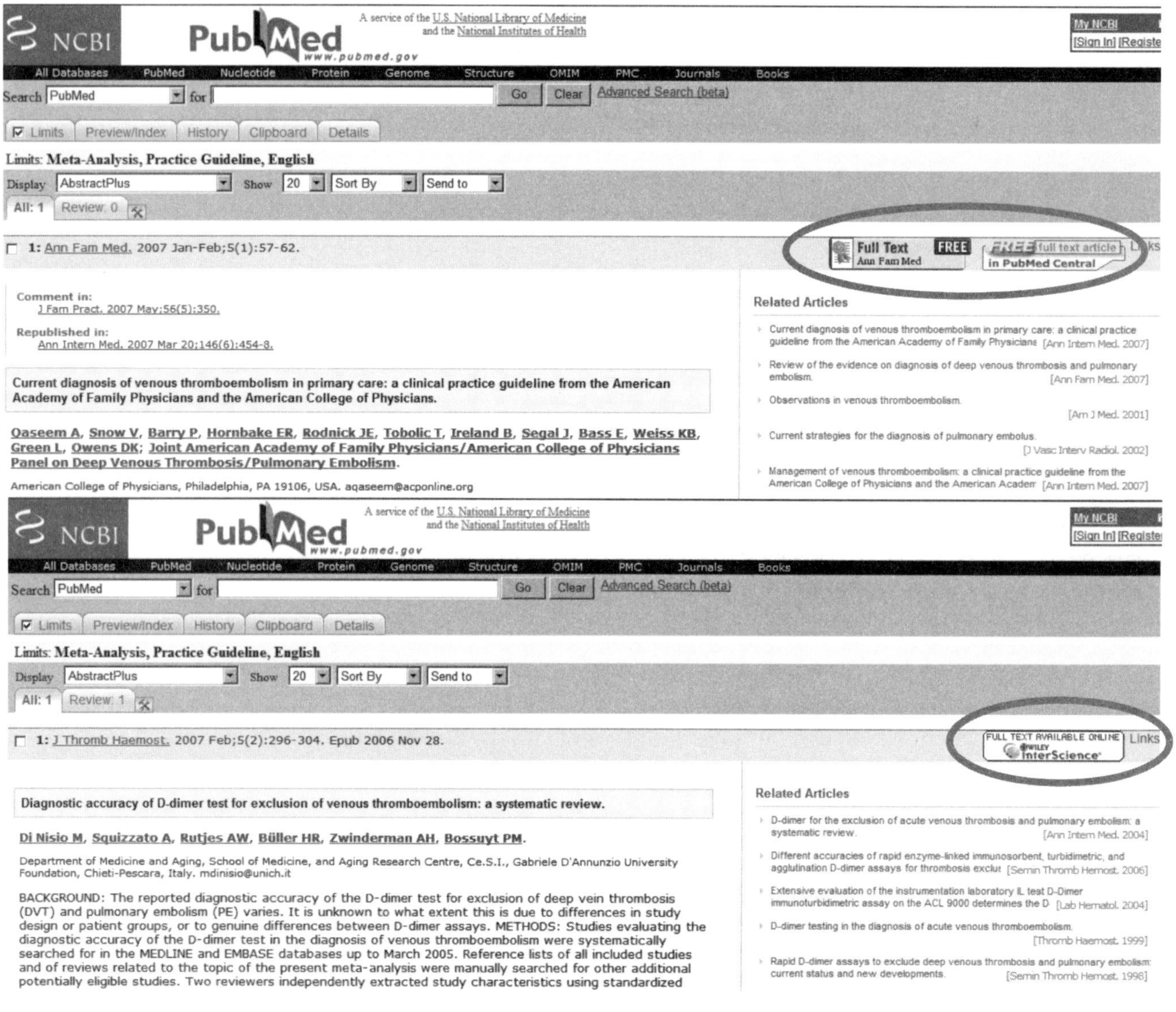

PubMed screen shot 11

Another useful tool for locating potentially relevant articles is the "Related Articles" function (PubMed screen shot 12). This function, located on the right-hand side of the PubMed page, can help find useful papers on similar topics—some of which are not found when using conventional searching strategies. By selecting any of the links, a separate PubMed page opens and displays the article with the abstract (if available), PDF (if available), and another set of related articles. By using this feature you can broaden your literature search as needed.

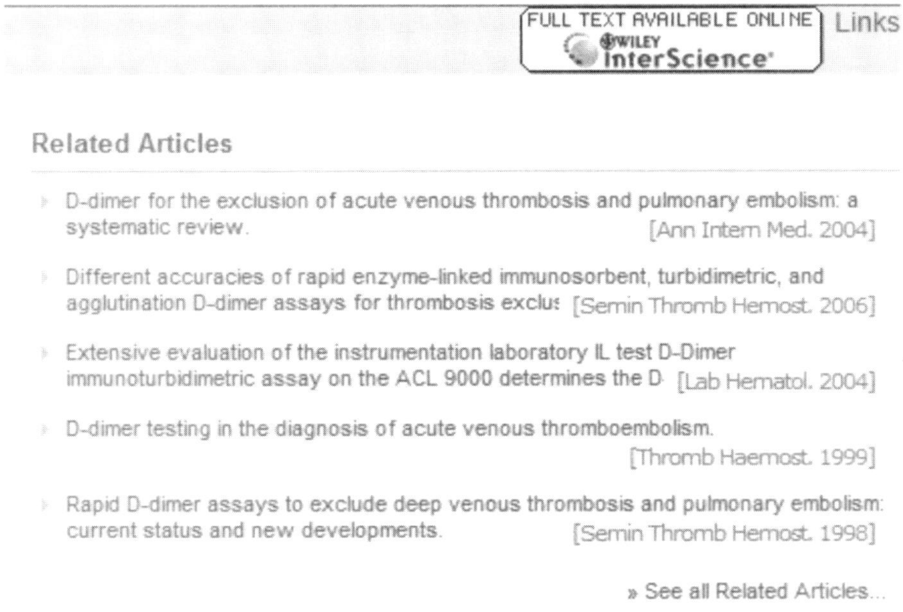

PubMed screen shot 12

Although the examples here have focused on MEDLINE and PubMed, other search resources are also available (refer to table on pages 95 and 96). Each has its own features, however the basic search logic, in general, is similar.

Pause and Reflect

Now apply what you've just learned to this problem:

You are contacted by a general practitioner in a multi-disciplinary patient care group that manages patients in the community with a high prevalence of congestive heart failure (CHF). He tells you that several groups are considering of the use of B-type natriuretic peptide (BNP) for guiding therapy in stabilized heart failure patients. You are aware that caring for patients with stable heart failure is complicated, particularly when patients are asymptomatic in spite of significant left ventricular

Continued

Pause and Reflect (Cont'd)

and diastolic dysfunction. You also know from experience that frequently patients with signs and symptoms of heart failure turn out to have optimized care for heart failure, and other co-morbidities account for their symptoms. He asks how strongly he should consider using BNP for guiding therapy in his stable (CHF) patients.

Population: ....

Intervention: ....

Comparator: ....

Outcome: ....

Using the PICO format, you formulate the following **question**:

....

....

Underline terms in the question above that will be important for your search.

Access PubMed on your computer at http://www.ncbi.nlm.nih.gov/sites/entrez/ (or www.pubmed.gov) and conduct the search.

Is congestive heart failure the best search term, or are there other MeSH terms that may yield better results?

....

....

Record your strategy

....

....

....

....

How many articles were retrieved? ....

Does it make a difference if the search is "narrow" versus "broad" for "Clinical Queries"?

....

....

....

Compare what you have recorded for your question, see the MeSH for heart failure, and compare the number of papers you retrieved with the following.

Question:

*Can **BNP** be used for guiding **therapy** in stable **CHF** patients?*

The MeSH hierarchy is shown in PubMed screen shot 13. It is better to use "Heart Failure" than the keyword "CHF" because "Heart Failure" is a broader term that includes many more terms that are relevant (PubMed screen shot 13). However, for this example try using a narrow search strategy, first using the term "Heart Failure" (screen shot 14), and then "Congestive Heart Failure." Does it make any difference?

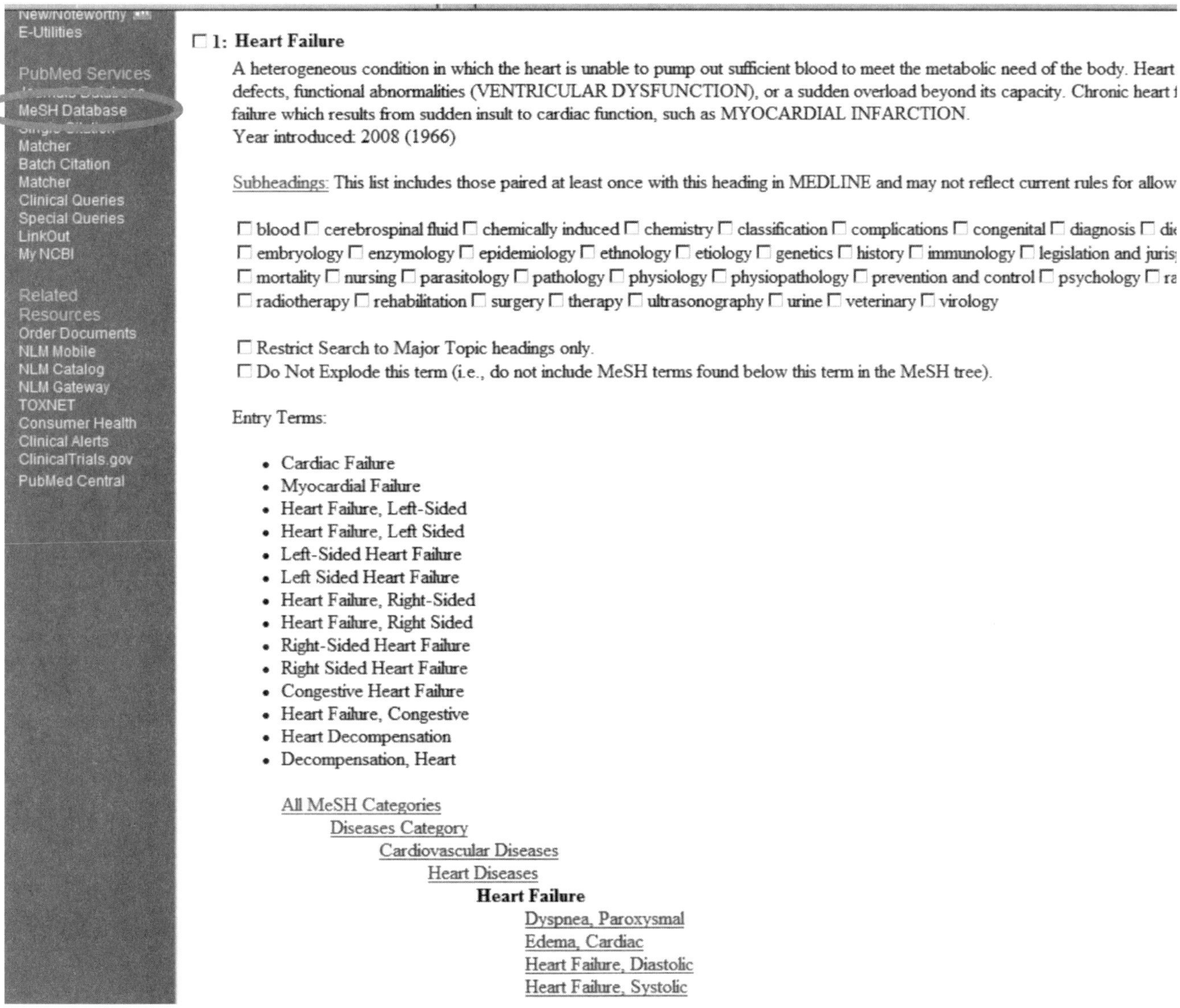

PubMed screen shot 13

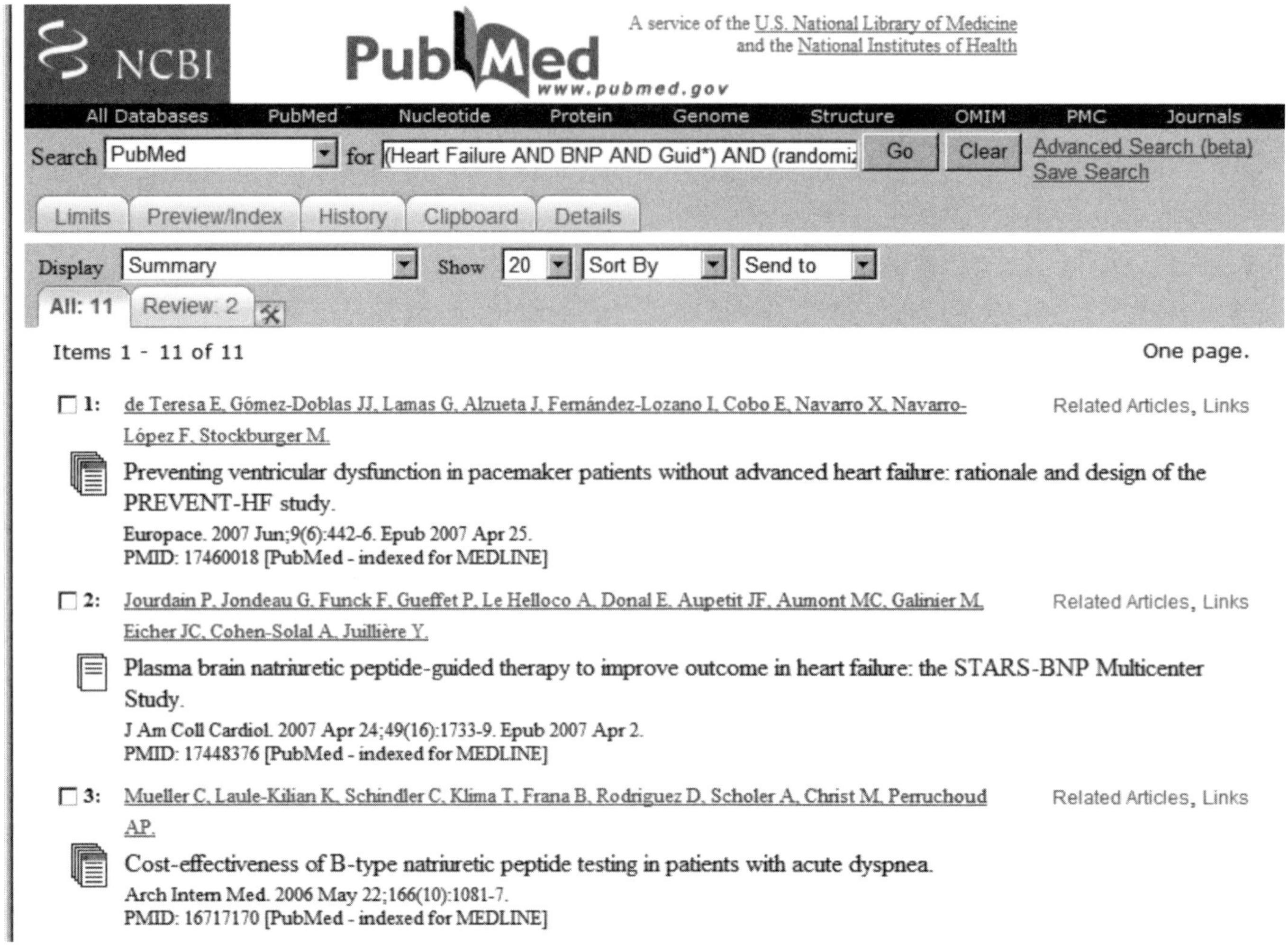

PubMed screen shot 14— Search terms = (Heart Failure AND BNP AND Guid*) AND (randomized controlled trial[Publication Type] OR (randomized[Title/Abstract] AND controlled[Title/Abstract] AND trial [Title/Abstract]))

Key Concept

Acquiring evidence is driven by the clinical question. Searching is often a dynamic process that utilizes various features of PubMed or any relevant database. Obtaining the assistance of a professional librarian can be essential in cases where comprehensive searching is necessary.

References

1. Brown MD, Lau J, Nelson RD, Kline JA. Turbidimetric D-dimer test in the diagnosis of pulmonary embolism: a metaanalysis. Clin Chem 2003;49:1846–53.

2. Klovning A, Sandberg S. Searching the literature. In: Price CP, Christenson RH, eds. Evidence-Based Laboratory Medicine: Principles, Practice, and Outcomes, 2nd ed. Washington, DC: AACC Press, 2007:189–212.

3. Watine J, Oosterhuis WP, Nagy E, et al. Formulating and using evidence-based guidelines. In: Price CP, Christenson RH, eds. Evidence-Based Laboratory Medicine: Principles, Practice, and Outcomes, 2nd ed. Washington, AACC Press, 2007:275–94.

STEP A3: APPRAISE—Critically Evaluate the Evidence

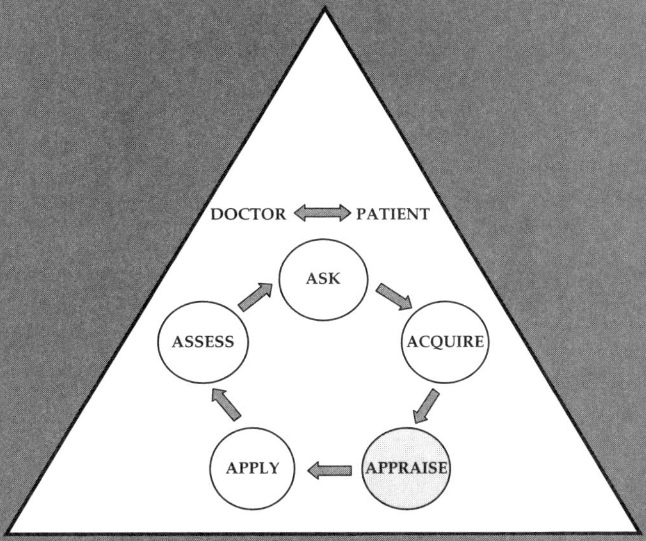

In this chapter

- An overview of the critical appraisal process
- Three fundamental questions for critically appraising evidence
- Key factors in the critical appraisal process
- Overview of tools for critical appraisal of studies (checklists) and for appraising quality of methodology (RAMMbo)
- Specific applications of different critical appraisal tools
- Step-by-step appraisal of diagnostic, prognostic, and outcome studies
- Critical appraisal of a technology
- Opportunities to practice and record a critical appraisal

Appraise: Critically Evaluating the Evidence

Appraisal of evidence is a fundamental part of the "A5 Cycle." In laboratory medicine, we use an organized protocol for evaluating foreground research evidence for relevance, validity, and practical use in decision making. Critical appraisal is essential to EBLM because "All that glitters is not gold." Most (even peer-reviewed) research is imperfect and/or does not exactly match the formulated clinical question(s).

Three Fundamental Questions

Critical appraisal is a structured approach that aids in maintaining focus on the primary clinical question. It also helps avoid wasting time or being distracted or misled by considering irrelevant or misinformation regarding

- **the relevance of the study's aim to the problem,**
- **appropriateness of the patient population,**
- **quality of the study's conduct or other important factors.**

Critical appraisal can also help the user gauge the difference between information of a theoretical nature and information gained from research trials and application in actual clinical practice.

Note that critical appraisal is frequently viewed as setting a very stringent standard; however it is important to realize that critical appraisal is not an exact science and at the "end of the day" users of information must decide for themselves if the available evidence is adequate and "close enough" for application to the question of interest.

What You'll Learn in This Section

In this chapter, you'll learn which features to look for in individual studies (primary research) and reviews (secondary research), so that critical appraisal can be performed consistently and efficiently in practice. Fortunately, simple tools that have been developed to assist with the critical appraisal process are readily available. These tools will be described and applied to a sample case later in the chapter.

Key Concept

Critical appraisal is a structured approach to evaluating evidence. This structured approach aids in maintaining focus on

- the primary clinical question,
- the relevance of evidence to the problem,
- potential biases such as appropriateness of the patient population, and
- quality of the study's conduct.

The Critical Appraisal Process: Key Factors

The success of the critical appraisal process relies on selecting "best evidence" to answer the clinical question (derived via PICO). This process itself involves evaluating the relevance of a study to your clinical question and being wary of confounders that can influence study results. It also involves evaluating study quality, paying attention to study design and possible sources of bias. All these factors are discussed in further detail below.

Selecting Best Evidence

Not all evidence is of equal quality. And unfortunately the literature and other sources of evidence can have a great deal of bias, the most serious of which is patient spectrum bias *(1, 2)* in which the study subjects do not match the target patient(s) in the context of the question being considered. Four levels of evidence (from least to most biased) can be classified according to type of research question (see Appendix B).

For all types of questions, the most reliable form of evidence is a systematic review—because these reviews represent a careful distillation of information for a specific question after vigilant measures are taken to assure transparency. Systematic reviews are developed using established protocols intended to mitigate subjectivity and to include the best-conducted and most reliable individual studies. Unfortunately, high quality systematic reviews have been conducted for relatively few topics in laboratory medicine.

Key Concept

For all types of questions, the most reliable form of evidence is a systematic review.

Making PICO the Key Focal Point

Just as in conducting clinical research, the clinical question must always remain the first task, driver, and focal point of critical appraisal—hence the importance of applying PICO when seeking an answer to that question.

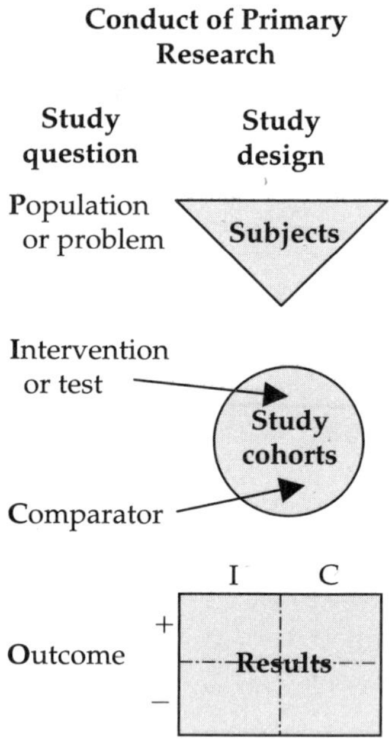

Evaluating Study Relevance

Once you've identified the clinical question (problem), then you'll evaluate the relevance of each phase of research to your clinical problem, for example,

- What's the question?
- Was the study conducted well methodologically?
- How reliable are the results?

Looked at this way, critical appraisal consists of thinking how the user would have designed the "ideal" study to answer the question, and then assess how well the primary or secondary research process matches the ideal (or improves on it).

Being Wary of Confounders

During critical appraisal the user must be alert for "confounders." Confounding factors are differences between cohorts that can cause test results to be misrepresented. Confounders commonly include age, gender, race, lifestyle, and socioeconomic status. There may well be many others, depending on the clinical question.

Age as a confounder
A typical example of a confounder is age. Suppose the outcome of interest for a test is 10-year mortality; one study group has a median age of 35 years while another has a median age of 85 years. Obviously one can guess which group will likely have higher mortality over the subsequent 10 years, pretty much regardless of the test result.

Focusing closely on the clinical question is critical for determining whether or not a particular characteristic for a study population is a confounder. For example, even with acutely ill patients who have the same disease or condition but are of different age groups, if the setting is the emergency department versus a primary care clinic comprised mainly of different ethnic groups, or critical care versus other locations in the hospital, or primary prevention versus secondary prevention involving clinics with different gender mixes, the study population can involve a different and possibly irrelevant spectrum of patients and confounders.

To assess possible confounders when you are evaluating evidence, carefully examine the patient characteristics and factors listed in the study's demographics table (usually "Table 1"). Evaluating how these possible characteristics match your clinical question will help determine confounders, and help focus on how they were accounted for in study design and adjustment.

Study design and methodology can help avoid confounders or they can be adjusted for statistically—but high-quality studies take measures to avoid the issue of confounders in their design and conduct.

Assessing Study Quality

The term "quality" can confer many meanings, including "degree or grade of excellence or worth." In the context of critical appraisal, overall quality is the extent to which scientific research is relevant, valid, complete, and applicable.

The biggest threat to quality is a "four-letter word"—*bias*. Bias results in poor evidence and a high risk of being misled by information from the searching (acquisition) process.

Be aware that appropriate trial design is the key to minimizing bias. Different trial designs are appropriate for addressing various types of clinical questions (see trial designs and levels of evidence in Appendix B and in the table in the Step A2 section, ACQUIRE—Find the Evidence, on page 92).

Sources of potential bias for diagnostic tests are listed in the glossary in Part 3; as noted earlier, spectrum bias can have the largest impact, as indicated in the figure below.

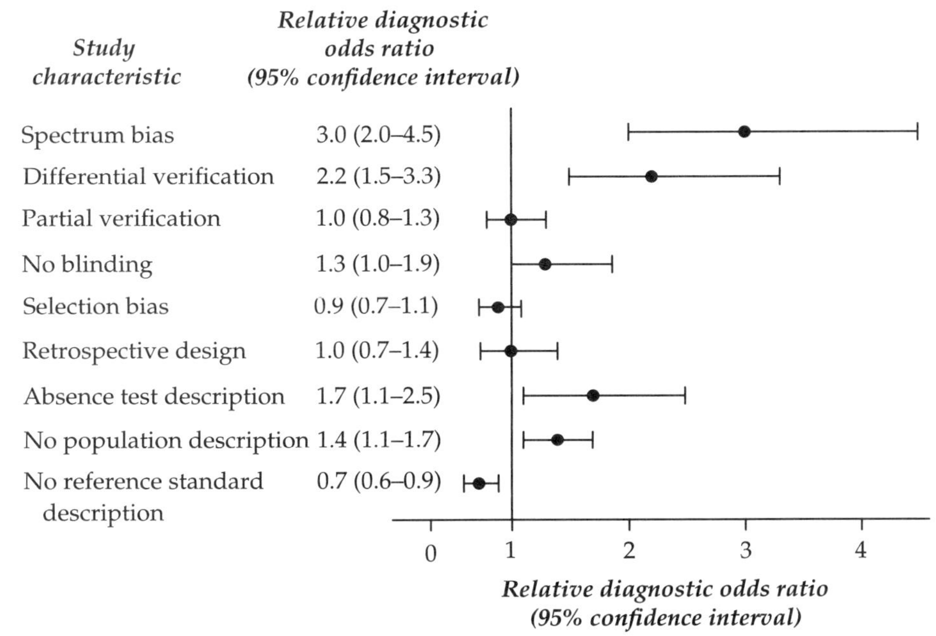

Reprinted with permission from Reference 2.

Gender (sex) as a confounder
Creatinine values are used for assessment of renal function; higher values are associated with renal insufficiency, i.e., lowered glomerular filtration rate (GFR). Because creatinine is a breakdown product of skeletal muscle, individuals with larger muscle mass have higher creatinine values independent of GFR. On average, men have substantially higher muscle mass than women and also, on average, higher creatinine values. For this reason, equations for estimating GFR have been developed that include gender as a variable to help minimize the differences in assessing renal function in men and women. Thus in studies for which renal function is an important variable and include both men and women, reporting only creatinine could be a confounder unless the gender appropriate estimated GFR values are reported also.

"BIAS" is the worst four-letter word in EBLM!

Appraising Individual Studies

There are three fundamental questions in the process of critically appraising primary or secondary studies:

(i) What is the PICO for the study; does it match closely enough to be relevant to your PICO?

(ii) How well was the study conducted?

(iii) What is the interpretation of the results and what is the uncertainty?

Once the literature base is identified and the initial search has eliminated irrelevant information, then initiate the critical appraisal process. Regardless of trial design, an efficient first step is to screen each study with questions oriented to the type of study question or issue addressed. For example, if the study is a

Systematic review:

Did the review ask a clearly focused question?
Did the review include the right types of studies?

Diagnostic test:
Was there a clear question for the study to address?
Was there comparison with an appropriate reference standard?

Cohort study (or case-control study):

Did the study address a clearly focused issue?
Did the authors use an appropriate method to answer their question?

Randomized controlled trial:

Did the study ask a clearly focused question?
Was this a randomized controlled trial (RCT) and was it randomized appropriately?

Regardless of trial design, a first screening issue involves clarity and focus of the clinical question. If the question or aim is not precisely stated or focused on the problem at hand, then the remaining information will be of modest benefit at best, so appraisal and inclusion of the report should go no further.

Key Concepts

- The most reliable form of evidence is a systematic review.
- The clinical question (as derived via PICO) must remain the key focal point of the critical appraisal process.
- Consider the "ideal" study design for your question—then assess how well the research you're reviewing matches the ideal. Be wary of confounders.
- In evaluating study quality, assess the extent to which the research is relevant, valid, complete, and applicable to your patient population.
- Be aware of potential bias, remembering that an appropriate trial design is the key to minimizing bias.

Tools for Critical Appraisal

Tools for critical appraisal of evidence consist of staged checklists. Checklists represent a simple, straightforward, and organized strategy for maintaining focus on any task—be it aeronautics (see sidebar) or EBLM.

Critical appraisal checklists necessarily vary somewhat according to the trial design. In the end, the essence of critical appraisal checklists is to vet study results, their applicability to the issue under consideration, and their minimization of bias regardless of the clinical question or trial design.

Some critical appraisal checklists, most of which have been developed by various stakeholder groups in EBM, are listed below, with a brief explanation of each.

Appraisal Checklists

1. **QUADAS: Qu**ality **A**ssessment of **D**iagnostic **A**ccuracy in **S**ystematic Reviews
   http://pubmedcentral.gov/articlerender.fcgi?artid=305345
   For use in performing systematic reviews to assess the quality of primary studies of diagnostic accuracy.
2. **CASP: C**ritical **A**ppraisal **S**kills **P**rogramme
   http://www.phru.nhs.uk/pages/PHD/resources.htm
   Developed by the Public Health Resource Unit (PHRU), a not-for-profit National Health Service public health consultancy in the United Kingdom. PHRU adapted critical appraisal tools for use in evaluating a variety of study types including diagnostic, economic, qualitative, randomized controlled trials, case control, and cohort studies, as well as systematic reviews.
3. **AGREE: A**ppraisal of **G**uidelines for **Re**search and **E**valuation
   http://www.agreecollaboration.org/
   A framework for assessing the quality of clinical practice guidelines developed through discussion among researchers having extensive experience and knowledge in clinical guidelines.
4. **STEP: S**creening and Diagnostic **T**est **E**valuation **P**rogram
   http://www.health.usyd.edu.au/step/
   For exploring the test performance characteristics of different screening and diagnostic tests. Part of a public health program to help evaluate and understand which screening programs are worthwhile and examine how those that are worthwhile should be best implemented.

Continued

On October 30, 1935, Boeing Corporation entered Model 299—a plane that could carry five times as many bombs as existing bombers and fly faster and twice as far—in a flight competition to determine which airplane manufacturer would build the next-generation long-range bomber.

Evaluators watched the plane taxi, lift, and climb to 300 feet. Then it stalled, turned, and crashed. Two crew members and the pilot died in the explosion.

The investigation blamed the crash on pilot error. He'd "... forgotten to release a new locking mechanism on the elevator and rudder controls." The newspapers called the Boeing model "too much airplane for one man to fly." Boeing faced near-certain bankruptcy.

The pilot had been a "top gun," so in all likelihood, requiring pilots to take more training didn't seem like the right response to the accident. Instead, Boeing took an incredibly simple approach: they created a pilot's checklist, with individual entries for takeoff, flight, landing, and taxiing.

Using the checklist became standard operating procedure. The results? "Pilots [flew] the Model 299 ... 1.8 million miles without one accident. The Army ultimately ordered almost 13,000 of the aircraft ... dubbed [it] the B-17, [and used it to gain] ... a decisive air advantage in the Second World War."

Source: "The Checklist." http://www.newyorker.com/reporting/2007/12/10/071210fa_fact_gawande (Accessed October 8, 2008).

Appraisal Checklists (Cont'd)

5. **CEBM:** Oxford **C**entre for **E**vidence **B**ased **M**edicine
   http://www.cebm.net/index.asp
   A number of appraisal forms for evaluating diagnostic, prognostic, evaluation of harm, therapeutic questions, and systematic reviews, developed by The Centre for Evidence-Based Medicine at Oxford. The site also contains useful definitions and calculators.

6. **CHE:** Canadian **C**entre for **H**ealth **E**vidence
   http://www.cche.net/usersguides/main.asp
   Variety of materials and check sheets including useful examples developed by the Centre for Health Evidence (CHE), a multi-disciplinary initiative that brings universities, health organizations, and professional associations together.

Although these checklists provide an excellent framework for assessing quality, some modification may be necessary for specific applications. CASP, for example, has perhaps the broadest scope; the program includes tools for critical appraisal of a wide variety of different studies, including economic, therapeutic, and diagnostic testing. Specifically, the CASP checklist covers items you should look for in a study (many of these items deal with bias). These items are included so that appraisers can separate useful literature from information that can be misleading.

Appraising Methodological Quality

RAMMbo is an aid for appraising the methodological quality of studies *(3)*. RAMMbo is an acronym:

- the **R** signifies "Recruitment," and reminds appraisers to check that the subjects represent the target population;
- the **A** signifies "Allocation or adjustment," and reminds the appraiser that, for example, consecutive enrollment is important for prognostic studies in order to avoid bias;
- the first **M** is for "Maintenance," and reminds the appraiser that the comparable status of the cohorts must be maintained;
- the second **M** is for "Measurement" reminding appraisers to ensure the outcomes were
  - **b**linded to the assessors, and
  - producing an **o**bjective outcome.

RAMMbo Evaluation of Study Methods

Fair **R**ecruitment	**R**	Recruit a large enough sample AND Recruit and randomize subjects OR Recruit consecutive patients
Fair **A**llocation - Comparable groups	**A**	Allocate randomly OR conceal allocations OR adjust for confounders (statistically or by matching)
Fair **M**aintenance	**M**	Manage groups equally. Follow up all subjects AND assess relevant outcomes in the starting groups
Fair **M**easurement - **b**linded (Valid/unbiased) - **o**utcome assessment	**M** **b** **o**	Measure outcomes with blinding of subjects and/or assessors AND/OR objective measures

Note that the acronym "RAAMbo" is used in other sources to signify the same concept *(4)*.

There is a clear relationship between the question formulated in PICO format and RAMMbo. RAMMbo deals almost entirely with methodological issues, not with fundamental relevance of the study to the clinical question. Keeping RAMMbo in mind when using the CASP (or any other) appraisal checklist helps maintain focus on items that are most important when appraising reliability of results.

Key Concept

Use a critical appraisal checklist to vet study results, their applicability to the issue under consideration, and their minimization of bias.

Critical Appraisal: Diagnostic and Prognostic Applications

Let's walk through an application of the appraisal process to questions of diagnosis and prognosis.

Clinical Laboratory Scenario

The "natriuretic peptide" test—i.e., either B-type Natriuretic Peptide (BNP) or Amino-terminal proBNP (NT-proBNP)—has evolved into having substantial importance for your emergency department staff. The test aids in the diagnostic assessment of patients presenting with dyspnea and also for prognostication of these patients, in part, to determine their venue of care, i.e., admission to the hospital, scheduling a follow-up outpatient appointment with cardiology, or sending them home.

You are considering some instrumentation that includes BNP and NT-proBNP. The emergency department staff trust your decision; however they have expressed particular concern about NT-proBNP, and whether the test will perform in patients with renal insufficiency. This is an important issue, as about 50% of the patients presenting with dyspnea have an estimated glomerular filtration rate (eGFR) <60 mL · minute^{-1} · (1.73 m^2)$^{-1}$.

Most of the primary studies in the literature have demonstrated that BNP and NT-proBNP tests perform virtually the same for use in diagnosis and prognosis in emergency department patients with dyspnea *(5, 6)*. However these earlier studies specifically excluded patients with impaired renal function; therefore the comparative performance of BNP and NT-proBNP in patients with eGFR <60 mL · minute^{-1} · (1.73 m^2)$^{-1}$ is uncertain to you.

From this scenario, two questions about comparative test performance are relevant for utilization in your emergency department population, one diagnostic and the other prognostic.

Diagnostic Application

Diagnostic question:

What is the relative performance of BNP and NT-proBNP for diagnosis of decompensated heart failure (DHF; also termed "congestive heart failure," [CHF]) in patients presenting to the emergency department with renal insufficiency [eGFR<60 mL · minute^{-1} · (1.73 m^2)$^{-1}$] and other risk factors?

Patient population: Patients presenting with dyspnea who have an eGFR <60 mL · $minute^{-1}$ · $(1.73\ m^2)^{-1}$

Intervention/Test: BNP and NT-proBNP

Comparator/Control: Reference method for determining DHF diagnosis

Outcome: Relative diagnostic performance of BNP and NT-proBNP

You locate a paper that appears to address your question *(7)*. A reprint of this paper is available free at <http://www.clinchem.org/cgi/reprint/53/8/1511>. Obtaining a copy of this paper will prove useful for the next exercise.

The next step is to work through the CASP checklist included as Appendix C. This specific checklist is designed for critical appraisal of diagnostic tests. Remember to keep in mind the RAMMbo methodological aspects.

Screening questions:

1. *Was there a clear question for the study to address?*

> The question should contain the population, the test, the reference standard, the setting, and the outcomes.

As stated in the introductory section of the paper, the authors *"... compared the diagnostic accuracy of NT-proBNP and BNP for diagnosing decompensated HF ... in ... patients with a full spectrum of impaired renal function who presented to a community hospital."*

Response: Yes

2. *Was there a comparison with an appropriate reference standard?*

> Is the reference test(s) the best available indicator in the circumstances?

In the "Materials and Methods" section of the paper, adjudication of each case was based on evaluation of a standard case report form for diagnosis of DHF by a cardiologist blinded to the NT-proBNP or BNP value. The blinding addresses the "b" aspect of RAMM<u>b</u>o. The method for determining eGFR was the four-variable Modification of Diet in Renal Disease formula.

Response: Yes

Is it worth continuing?

Response: Yes; the response to both screening questions is yes.

3. *Did all the patients get the diagnostic test and reference standard?*

Look for verification bias (see Part 3 Glossary).

In the "Materials and Methods" section, it was stated that all patients received NT-proBNP and BNP testing; a case report form was completed and all subjects were adjudicated to determine whether the diagnosis was DHF.

Receiver operating characteristic (ROC) curve analysis was performed and diagnostic sensitivity, specificity, accuracy, and negative and positive predictive values were reported.

Response: Yes. The "Measurement" aspect of RAM**M**bo was appropriate.

4. *Could results for the test of interest have been influenced by the results of the reference standard?*

Was there blinding? Were the tests performed independently? Look for review bias [Part 3 Glossary].

In the Methods section, it was noted that the adjudicating cardiologist was blinded to the NT-proBNP and BNP values.

Response: Blinding was part of the study design. The blinding aspect of RAMM**b**o was appropriate.

5. *Is the disease status of the tested population clearly described?*

Note presenting symptoms, disease stage or severity, co-morbidity, and differential diagnostics. Is there any evidence of spectrum bias?

In Table 1 and "Materials and Methods" it was noted that the patients were consecutive. Table 1 of the study shows the age, gender, race, body mass index, and overall NT-proBNP and BNP values along with other characteristics broken out by eGFR either $>$ or $<$60 mL · minute^{-1} · (1.73 m^2)$^{-1}$.

Response: The spectrum of patients included in the study closely matches the question. The consecutive patients and fair "Allocation" and "Recruitment" aspects of **RA**MMbo were covered.

6. *Were the methods for performing the test described in sufficient detail? Was a protocol followed?*

Was a protocol followed?

The methods were well described for the patients included in the study. A protocol was followed systematically with no apparent verification or review bias. However, the possibility of spectrum bias must be kept in mind due to the relevance of renal insufficiency in your patient population. The "Measurement" aspects of RAM**M**bo are appropriate.

Is it worth continuing?

Response: Yes

7. *What are the results?*

Are sensitivity and specificity and/or likelihood ratios presented?

Specific values for patients with eGFR <60 mL · minute^{-1} · (1.73 m^2)$^{-1}$ and >60 mL · minute^{-1} · (1.73 m^2)$^{-1}$ were reported with ROC areas. Diagnostic sensitivity, specificity, and positive and negative predictive values were reported for NT-proBNP and BNP at appropriate decision points.

Response: The results were reported in a useful way.

8. *How sure are we about these results?*

Could the results have occurred by chance? Are there confidence limits? What are they?

The number of patients included in the trial was 831. Confidence limits were reported and were quite narrow, providing evidence that the study was powered properly. The likelihood that the results occurred by chance is low.

9. *Can the results be applied to your patients/the population of interest?*

Do you think your patient(s) differ(s) from those in the study such that the results cannot be applied? Consider age, sex, ethnicity, and the possibility of spectrum bias.

The results can be generalized to the patient population in your question. NT-proBNP and BNP showed very similar characteristics for diagnosis of DHF regardless of renal function.

10. *Can the test be applied to your patient or the population of interest?*

Consider resources, opportunity costs, level and availability of expertise required for interpretation, and current practice and availability of services.

NT-proBNP and BNP measurements are readily available (costs to be determined by negotiation with instrument vendor). Interpretation of NT-proBNP might be viewed as more complicated in patients with eGFR >60 mL · minute^{-1} · (1.73 m^2)$^{-1}$. However, in patients with eGFR <60 mL · minute^{-1} · (1.73 m^2)$^{-1}$, a single cutoff of >1200 ng/L is appropriate for NT-proBNP and a single cutoff of >200 ng/L for BNP. Diagnostic performance is not different for these natriuretic peptides.

Response: The markers are not different for DHF diagnosis in patients with eGFR <60 mL · minute^{-1} · (1.73 m^2)$^{-1}$.

11. *Were all outcomes important to the individual or population considered?*

Comparative diagnostic performance of NT-proBNP and BNP was the primary outcome. Other outcomes such as all-cause mortality were considered, and change in patient management based on either result would most probably be impacted. However differences in management based on BNP or NT-proBNP was not specifically investigated in this study.

Will knowledge of BNP or NT-proBNP improve patient well-being? Will knowledge of the test results lead to a change in patient management?

12. *What would be the impact of using this test on your patients/population?*

The decision of which instrument platform to use can be made independent of natriuretic peptide. Either NT-proBNP or BNP is effective for diagnosis of DHF regardless of renal function, provided the appropriate cut-points are utilized.

Consider whether you use either test based on the evidence.

Key Concepts

This critical appraisal has determined affirmative responses; the report addressed a head-to-head comparison of NT-proBNP and BNP in a population with 47% renal insufficiency patients, typical for community hospital populations. The paper reports ROC curve areas and diagnostic performance at relevant decision points, all with 95% confidence intervals. Therefore, the results appear to be close enough to help with answering the question about the diagnostic testing.

Prognostic Application

It turns out that this same paper followed patients for a median of 400 days after the first presentation with dyspnea. Thus the same paper *(7)* will be used to assess prognostic use of BNP and NT-proBNP.

Prognostic question:

What is the relative prognostic performance of BNP and NT-proBNP in patients with dyspnea and other risk factors, including renal insufficiency [eGFR <60 mL · minute^{-1} · (1.73 m^2)$^{-1}$], who present to the emergency department?

Patient population: Patients presenting to emergency department with dyspnea and other risk factors including a continuum of renal function.

Intervention/Test: BNP and NT-proBNP

Comparator/Control: Either none, or patients with relatively lower BNP and NT-proBNP values

Outcome: Ability of BNP and NT-proBNP to predict adverse event(s)

According to the table in Step A2, page 92), the appropriate type of study for assessing prognosis is a cohort study. Thus, the next step is to work through the CASP appraisal checklist designed for cohort (prognostic) studies; this is included as Appendix D. Again, keep in mind the methodological items from RAMMbo.

Screening questions:

1. *Did the study address a clearly focused issue?*

   See the introductory section of the paper: The authors "*. . . compared . . . NT-proBNP and BNP for . . . predicting 1-year all-cause mortality in . . . patients with a full spectrum of impaired renal function who presented to a community hospital.*"

   Response: Yes. The prognostic outcome was alive or dead from any cause. They attempted to detect a good or bad outcome with NT-proBNP or BNP measurements.

The question should contain the population, the risk factors, and outcome considered. It should be clear that the study attempted to detect a good or bad prognostic effect.

2. *Did the authors use an appropriate method to answer their question?*

   An inception cohort study is an appropriate design for addressing prognostic questions. All patients had dyspnea on presentation and all presented to an emergency department at inception.

   Response: Yes.

Is a cohort study a valid way of answering this prognostic question? Did it address the study question?

Is it worth continuing?

Response: Yes. It is worth continuing with the critical appraisal.

3. *Was the cohort recruited in an acceptable way?*

   The Materials and Methods section indicates that consecutive patients were included in the study. Table 1 from the paper shows that 47% of the cohort had eGFR <60 mL · minute^{-1} · (1.73 m^2)$^{-1}$; this renal insufficiency prevalence is similar to that in your emergency department. Further, there was a spectrum of renal insufficiency in that 16.7% of the population had eGFR values of <30 mL · minute^{-1} · (1.73 m^2)$^{-1}$.

   Response: The cohort was recruited in an acceptable way. The "Recruitment" aspect of **R**AMMbo is appropriate.

Selection bias could compromise the study and must be avoided. Was the cohort representative of the appropriate population or was it "special" in some way? Was everybody included who should have been included?

4. *Was the exposure accurately measured to minimize bias?*

   BNP and NT-proBNP measurements are objective and reflect what will be encountered in laboratory medicine practice. The measurements for both are continuous variables that allow classification of patients with dyspnea using the same procedure. The patients were allocated according to the magnitude of their BNP or NT-proBNP values.

   Response: Yes. The "Allocation" aspect of RAMMbo was appropriate.

> Were measurements (BNP and NT-proBNP) subjective or objective? Did they reflect what you want, and were subjects classified into groups using the same procedure?

5. *Was the outcome accurately measured to minimize bias?*

   The 1-year all-cause mortality outcome was objective; it was determined from the social security death index. Outcome status was determined in 98% of the cohort.

   Response: The outcome was objective and accurately measured.

> Were the outcomes subjective or objective and meaningful? Was a reliable and consistent system used for establishing and detecting outcomes for the cases? Were the measurement methods similar in the different groups? Was the outcome adjudicator blinded to the exposure (BNP and NT-proBNP)?

6. A. *Have the authors identified all the important confounding factors? List the ones that might be important, that the authors missed.*

   B. *Have they taken into account confounding factors in the design and/or analysis?*

   A. Important confounding factors including age, sex, race/ethnicity, eGFR, dialysis treatment, hypertension, diabetes, atrial fibrillation, coronary disease, prior heart failure, patient disposition, and diagnosis of DHF were accounted for. Other possible confounding factors were (i) performed at a single site; (ii) even though the Social Security Death Index is an acceptable method for determining death status, the exact cause of death remains unknown without case-by-case adjudication.

   B. These confounders were taken into account to the extent possible.

> Were confounders adequately considered? Look for restriction in design and techniques, e.g., modeling and stratified, regression, or sensitivity analysis to correct, control, or adjust for confounding factors.

   Response: Confounding factors were selected *a priori* and adjusted for by multivariate logistic regression. The potential confounders for which the study compensated included age, sex, race, renal function, history of dialysis treatment, diabetes, atrial fibrillation, hypertension, coronary artery disease, prior history of HF, and whether the patient was discharged to home or was admitted to a hospital ward or intensive care unit. The multivariate logistic regression approach was examined by evaluating the goodness of fit, which was reasonable. It is not possible to compensate for inclusion of a single site, but confounders were taken into account to the extent possible.

7. A. *Was the follow-up of subjects complete enough?*

   B. *Was the follow-up of subjects long enough?*

   Follow-up for the outcome of alive versus dead was 98%; the length of follow-up was 400 days (interquartile range 300–475 days).

   Response: Generally, follow-up of >90% is considered adequate. Knowledge of the typical mortality of the disease question and examining data from Kaplan-Meier curves can add insight into determining if follow-up is long enough. All-cause mortality over five years was about 80% for patients with HF. The Kaplan-Meier curves for the study dropped rather quickly in the first few months, and then appeared to flatten after about 10 months. This information helps indicate that the follow up was relatively complete and the follow-up long enough.

Assure that patient follow-up was appropriate (usually considered >90%). The good and bad effects should have had long enough to reveal themselves. The persons lost to follow-up may have different outcomes than those available for assessment.

8. *What are the results of the study?*

   Median NT-proBNP and BNP concentrations were 4.3-fold and 2.0-fold higher for subjects who died compared with those who survived, respectively. After adjusting for age, sex, race/ethnicity, eGFR, dialysis treatment, hypertension, diabetes, atrial fibrillation, coronary disease, prior heart failure, and patient disposition and diagnosis of DHF, patients in the upper quartile of values had a hazard ratio of 2.6 (95% CI: 1.4–4.8) for BNP and 4.5 (95% CI: 2.0–10.2) for NT-proBNP compared to those in the lowest quartiles for the biomarkers. The hazard ratio for NT-proBNP was almost two-fold higher than BNP and appears to be a superior indicator of mortality.

What are the bottom-line results? Have the authors reported the rate or proportion between the higher/lower BNP and NT-proBNP values and the ratio or the rate difference?

9. *How precise are the results? How precise is the estimate of the risk?*

   Increasing values of both BNP and NT-proBNP showed a significant association with increasing risk of death after adjustment

Consider size of the confidence intervals.

for important variables including eGFR (P = 0.004 and P<0.001, respectively). The confidence intervals for the hazard ratio were 2.6 (95% CI: 1.4–4.8) for BNP and 4.5 (95% CI: 2.0–10.2) for NT-proBNP after adjustment for variables including age, sex, race/ethnicity, eGFR, dialysis treatment, hypertension, diabetes, atrial fibrillation, coronary disease, prior heart failure, patient disposition, and diagnosis of DHF.

Response: The results were quite precise.

10. *Do you believe the results?*

Consider items such as size of effect, reliability with regard to bias or confounding of results, time sequence, dose response gradient, and biological plausibility.

The study is relatively large (n=831), matches well with your population with respect to renal insufficiency and other variables, was performed in a community setting, and the findings are biologically plausible.

Response: The results are believable.

11. *Can the results be applied to the local population?*

Are the subjects sufficiently different from your population to cause concern? Is your local setting likely to differ from the study population?

There are many similarities with the local population, and technology for the testing is available.

Response: The results are close enough for application to the local population.

12. *Do the results of the study fit with other available evidence?*

Smaller studies have shown that increased BNP or NT-proBNP concentrations are highly predictive of mortality in patients with DHF and impaired renal function. Comparisons between BNP and NT-proBNP in the stable HF population for all-cause mortality showed a similarity between the two markers. Although these other studies did not match this problem as closely, the results are consistent with other studies.

Response: The results are consistent.

Critical Appraisal: Impact on Outcomes

The following is a critical appraisal exercise for assessing the impact of laboratory testing on outcomes. A CASP checklist for outcome studies is included in Appendix E. The clinical question is specified, but it is left to you to complete the exercise. After you have completed the exercise, you can compare your responses to a "worked–through" example in Appendix F. Remember to keep in mind the RAMMbo methodology.

Laboratory Medicine Scenario

One of the diabetologists in the hospital wishes to have a real time HbA1c result available when he sees his patients, believing that it may help him to manage his patients more effectively by giving immediate feedback on the results. He is aware that there are point-of-care testing (POCT) systems available that could be used in his clinic, and he wants to know if there is any evidence to support his contention that providing the test result in his clinic may lead to improved outcomes. The diabetologist is also aware of the trend toward managing patients with long-term conditions in the community setting, and wonders aloud as to whether such a clinic practice could be transferred into the community.

This conversation identifies two clear questions. In the first instance, suppose you agree to focus on the question in secondary care, while recognizing that, on the face of it, the two questions only appear to differ in terms of the setting in which care is delivered. Then you formulate the following question:

Will the measurement of HbA1c at the point of care (with immediate feedback of the results) lead to improved health outcomes, i.e., glycemic control, in the case of diabetics being managed in a secondary care setting? The health outcome needs to be defined explicitly (e.g., clinical, operational, or economic) and in this situation the diabetologist was interested in improved glycemic control and specifically HbA1c as a surrogate marker of long-term glycemic control.

You are aware that the National Academy of Clinical Biochemistry (NACB) Laboratory Medicine Practice Guidelines on POCT includes a section on the diagnosis and management of diabetes. This section covers the use of POCT for HbA1c measurement *(8)*, and subsequently there was a narrative update published *(9)*. You find a paper that you feel might address the question being asked *(10)*. This paper is available free at http://care.diabetesjournals.org/cgi/reprint/22/11/1785. Obtaining a copy of this paper will prove useful for the next exercise.

Patient population: ....

Intervention/Test: ....

Comparator/Control: ....

Outcome: ....

The CASP critical appraisal form for an outcome study is included in Appendix E. Items from the checklist are listed below for use in this exercise.

Screening questions:

1. *Was there a clear question for the study to address?*

   Response:

   ....

   ....

   ....

> The question should contain the population, the intervention (test), the control (test), the setting and the outcome.

2. *Was the intervention compared with a control group in a way that minimized bias, and yet ensured that the results were used to make clinical decisions leading to an outcome?*

   Response:

   ....

   ....

   ....

> Was the study a randomized controlled trial (as this is the best approach to minimizing bias)? (Note: It has been suggested that a before-and-after study design would be an alternative approach to testing the impact of diagnostic tests on health outcomes.)

Is it worth continuing?

Response: ....

3. *Were participants clearly identified and appropriately allocated to intervention and control groups?*

Response:

....

....

....

Intention-to-treat analysis is intended to avoid misrepresentation in intervention research studies. Intention to treat is based on the subject's initial assignment, not on the intervention actually administered. For the purpose of intention-to-treat analysis, all subjects who are assigned to receive the intervention are considered to be part of the trial and their outcomes count, whether they drop out or not.

4. *Were participants, staff, and study personnel "blind" to participant's study group?*

Response:

....

....

....

Was there blinding? (Look for observer or operator bias [Part 3 Glossary].)

5. *Were all of the participants who entered the trial accounted for at its conclusion?*

Response:

....

....

....

Results of the intervention group can be misleading if subjects who have a lower response to the intervention or a more serious disease drop out of the study at a higher rate, because then only the subjects assigned to the intervention group for whom the treatment worked will be analyzed. Thus ineffective interventions may appear to provide benefit if only the intervention subjects who finish the study are compared with controls.

This is why all the participants who entered the trial must be accounted for at its conclusion.

6. *Were the methods for performing the tests described, enough participants recruited, participants followed up, and data collected in the same way?*

Response:

....

....

....

> (i) Was a protocol followed for both the intervention and control arms?
>
> (ii) Were sufficiently robust outcome measures employed in the study?
>
> (iii) Was there a power calculation?
>
> (iv) Were all participants tested and monitored in the same way, at the same time intervals?

Is it worth continuing?

Response: ....

7. *How are the results presented and what is the main result?*

Response:

....

....

....

> (i) Were the correct statistical tools used?
>
> (ii) Are the results presented in such a way that we can work them out?
>
> (iii) How large is the size of the result and is it meaningful?

8. *How precise are these results?*

Response:

....

....

....

> (i) Is the result precise enough to make a decision?
>
> (ii) Are confidence limits reported?
>
> (iii) Are p-values reported?

9. *Can the results be applied to your patients/the population of interest?*

Response:

....

....

....

> (i) Do you think your patients/population are so different from those in the study that the results cannot be applied? (Hint: Consider age, sex, ethnicity, and spectrum bias.)
>
> (ii) Is your patient/population setting different from that of the trial, e.g., primary vs. secondary care?

10. *Can the test be applied to your patient or population of interest?*

Response:

....

....

....

Consider resources and opportunity costs, training, QA requirements, and expertise needed for test interpretation, and availability of services.

11. *Were all outcomes important to the individual or population considered?*

Response:

....

....

....

(i) Will knowledge of the test results improve patient well-being?

(ii) Will this knowledge of the test results lead to a change in patient management?

(iii) Will it be possible to make the required change in patient management?

(iv) Were any risks associated with adopting the approach taken in the trial explored and are they relevant to your situation?

12. *What would be the impact of using this test on your patients/population?*

Response:

....

....

....

You can now compare your responses to those in the worked-through example in Appendix F. This critical appraisal determined some affirmative responses to the question that was asked. There were also some difficult issues surrounding the performance of studies to assess the impact of diagnostic tests on patient outcomes. However, the appraisal also identified that changes must be made to clinical practice in order to deliver healthcare benefits through improved outcomes using a more effective care pathway.

Critical Appraisal of a Technology Systematic Review

Now read the scenario below and complete the appraisal process, starting with formulating the clinical question. A meta-analysis (systematic review) is available at no cost at http://www.clinchem.org/cgi/reprint/49/11/1846 *(11)*. Obtaining a copy of this paper will prove useful for the next exercise.

Laboratory Medicine Scenario

Your emergency department chair has approached you about offering D-dimer test for the work-up of pulmonary embolism and deep vein thrombosis in symptomatic patients presenting to their service. She points out that a number of colleagues at other medical centers in the area have implemented ELISA-type tests for this application. You have no ELISA-type technology for D-dimer measurements available in your laboratory currently and therefore may have to justify purchase of a dedicated system for this testing. You currently offer D-dimer by a quantitative latex turbidimetric testing method. You have been told that there are no more funds for new equipment. Is it really necessary to procure an instrument capable of ELISA-type D-dimer measurement, or will your qualitative latex turbidimetric test do for this purpose?

The first step is to formulate the clinical question and apply it to the PICO format.

P ....

I ....

C ....

O ....

The next task is to critically appraise, using the CASP checklist that follows, the systematic review that examines use of latex turbidimetric measurements for diagnosis of pulmonary embolism by Brown et al. *(11)*.

Appraisal of a Systematic Review*

1. *Did the review ask a clearly focused question?*

   Response:

   ....

> Consider if the question was "focused" in terms of
> - the population studied
> - the intervention given, or exposure
> - the outcomes considered

2. *Did the review include the right type of study?*

   Response:

   ....

> Consider if the review included studies that
> - address the review's question
> - have an appropriate study design

3. *Did the reviewers try to identify all of the relevant studies?*

   Response:

   ....

> Consider:
> - the bibliographic databases used
> - if there was follow-up from reference lists
> - if there was personal contact with experts
> - if the reviewers searched for unpublished studies
> - if the reviewers searched for non-English-language studies

4. *Did the reviewers assess the quality of the included studies?*

   Response:

   ....

> Consider:
> - a scoring system
> - more than one assessor

5. *If the results of the studies have been combined, was it reasonable to do so?*

   Response:

   ....

> Consider:
> - if the results of each study were clearly displayed
> - if the results were similar from study to study (look for heterogeneity)
> - if the reasons for any variations in results were discussed

6. *How are the results presented and what is the main result?*

Response:

....

> Consider:
> - how the results were expressed (odds ratio, negative risk, etc.)
> - how large, and how meaningful, the effect was
> - how you would sum up the bottom-line result or the review in one sentence

7. *How precise are the results?*

Response:

....

> Consider:
> - If confidence intervals (CIs) were reported, would your decision about whether or not to use this test be the same at the upper CI as the lower CI?
> - Is a p-value reported where CIs are unavailable?

8. *Can the results be applied to the local population?*

Response:

....

> Consider whether:
> - the population sample covered by the review could be different from your population in ways that would produce different results
> - your local setting differs much from that of the review
> - you can provide the same intervention in your setting

9. *Were all important outcomes considered?*

Response:

....

> Consider outcomes from the viewpoint of the
> - individual
> - policymakers and professionals
> - family/caregivers
> - wider community

10. *Should policy or practice change as a result of the evidence contained in this review?*

Response:

....

> Consider:
> - whether any benefit reported outweighs any harm and/or cost. If this information is not reported, can it be filled in from elsewhere?

References

1. Ransohoff DF, Feinstein AR. Problems of spectrum and bias in evaluating the efficacy of diagnostic tests. N Engl J Med 1978;299:926–30.
2. Lijmer JG, Mol BW, Heisterkamp S, et al. Empirical evidence of design-related bias in studies of diagnostic tests. JAMA 1999;282:1061–6.
3. Glasziou P, Del Mar C, Salisbury J. Evidence-Based Practice Workbook, 2nd ed. Oxford: Blackwell Publishing BMJ Books, 2007:202pp.
4. Jackson R, Ameratunga S, Broad J, et al. The GATE frame: critical appraisal with pictures. ACP Journal Club 2006;144;A8–A11.
5. Maisel AS, Krishnaswamy P, Nowak RM, et al. Rapid measurement of B-type natriuretic peptide in the emergency diagnosis of heart failure. N Engl J Med 2002;347:161–7.
6. Januzzi JL Jr, Camargo CA, Anwaruddin S, et al. The N-terminal Pro-BNP investigation of dyspnea in the emergency department (PRIDE) study. Am J Cardiol 2005;95:948–54.
7. deFilippi CR, Seliger SL, Maynard S, Christenson RH. Impact of renal disease on natriuretic peptide testing for diagnosing decompensated heart failure and predicting mortality. Clin Chem 2007;53:1511–9.
8. Aarsand AK, Alter D, Frost SJ, et al. Diagnosis and management of diabetes mellitus. In: Nichols JH, ed. The National Academy of Clinical Biochemistry Laboratory Medicine Practice Guidelines: Evidence-Based Practice for Point-of-Care Testing. Washington DC: AACC Press, 2006:44–62.
9. Price CP, Alter D, Sacks DB, et al. Point-of-care testing in the diagnosis and management of diabetes; a narrative update to the NACB guidelines. Point of Care 2007;6:237–42.
10. Cagliero E, Levina E, Nathan D. Immediate feedback of HbA1c levels improves glycemic control in type 1 and insulin-treated type 2 diabetic patients. Diabetes Care 1999;22:1785–9.
11. Brown MD, Lau J, Nelson RD, Kline JA. Turbidimetric D-dimer test in the diagnosis of pulmonary embolism: a metaanalysis. Clin Chem 2003;49:1846–53.

STEP A4: APPLY—Apply the Evidence to Your Clinical Situation

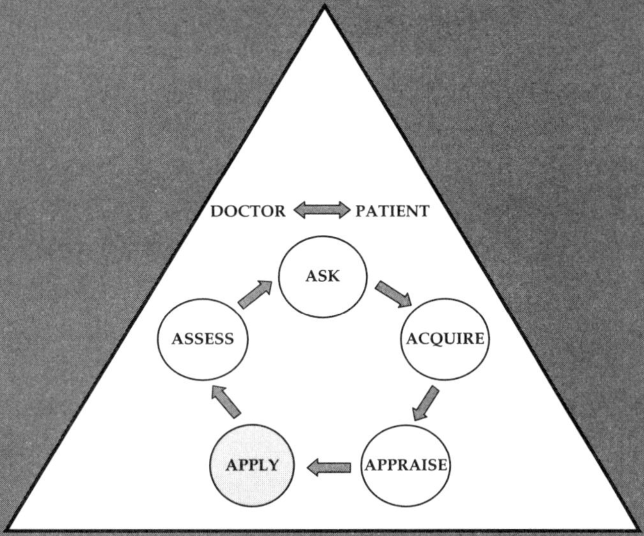

In this chapter

- Issues concerned with applying evidence to your clinical problem
- The hierarchy of evidence for clinical decision making
- Internal vs. external validity
- A generic checklist for applying evidence
- Sample applications to practice
- Taking stock of what you've learned
- Summary: applying evidence in practice

Apply: Applying the Evidence to Your Clinical Situation

When you believe you've located and appraised the evidence that will answer the question that was asked, you must think about the issues concerned with applying the evidence:

(i) **Patient or population:** Does the evidence apply to the patient or population referred to in the original question?

(ii) **Intervention:** Is the performance of the analytical method described, is the performance satisfactory for the applications described, and does my method have the required performance?

(iii) **Comparison or control:** Was there an adequate control method or comparison group (which may be a comparison with current practice or with best practice)?

(iv) **What change in clinical practice** is implicit in the application of the evidence (e.g., use of a new test, an alternative delivery method, etc.)?

(v) **Outcomes:** What outcomes are either demonstrated or claimed in the evidence presented? Can they be achieved?

To apply evidence effectively when resolving a problem requires understanding the question properly, ensuring that there is good evidence to support the change, and being aware of the changes in practice that will be required to deliver a good solution.

The hierarchy for test utilization on which one might make the decision to invest in the use of a test is illustrated here.

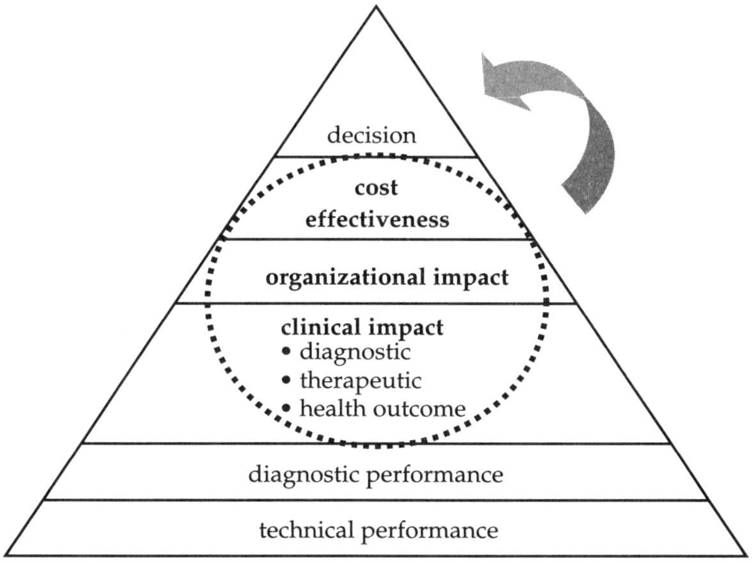

The hierarchy for test utilization required in laboratory medicine to make valid decisions on whether to buy or use a given diagnostic test. The key components to considering the health outcome are highlighted in the circle *(1)*

Modified from reference (1) with permission.

You see immediately that the core structure of PICO, employed in all of the previous steps, is relevant to applying the data. Furthermore, it is important to ensure that you use good quality evidence. There is also the challenge of the change management required to deliver the improvements expected from application of the evidence.

Internal vs. External Validity

When assessing a paper one looks for evidence of "internal validity" and of "external validity":

- **Internal validity** is concerned with ensuring that the design of the study described in the paper is robust and that every effort has been made to minimize the effects of systematic error or bias.
- **External validity** is concerned with the generalizability of the findings and whether the study has been conducted in accordance with methodological practice *(2)*.

In this section we address the issues concerned with "external validity"; this will help to determine whether the evidence you have found will be applicable to the problem you have to deal with (i.e., the clinical question that is being asked).

Key Concept

Whatever the claimed utility (utilities) for the test, it is important to be able to answer the last question in Sackett and Haynes' "The Architecture of Diagnostic Research" *(3)*—namely, "Do patients undergoing the diagnostic test fare better than similar untested patients?" Any application of evidence will always culminate in this question, whether the question concerns evaluating diagnostic performance, prognosis, monitoring, or health outcomes. There is little point in performing a test unless there is the potential for benefit—whether it be clinical, operational, or economic.

Note that studies on etiology and risk factors involve background knowledge and have less to do with answering the question of whether patients fare better; however, this background knowledge can be helpful.

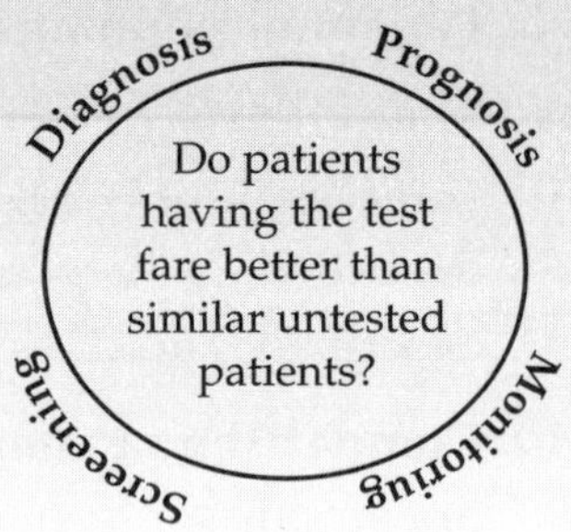

The key objective when offering a diagnostic test—whatever the application.

A Generic Checklist for Applying Evidence

In seeking to apply the information gained from a study, consider the following questions. Note that they are generic and not all of the questions are relevant to every application.

P: Is the patient (or population) similar to that described in the study?

- Does the patient (or population) with whom you are now concerned match those described in the study? Important factors to consider: age, sex, ethnicity, stage in the evolution of the condition, severity of condition.
- Are the patients (or population) featured in the study so different from those with whom you are concerned that the study results are not applicable to your population or patient?
- Is the setting of the study comparable to the setting in question (e.g., primary or secondary care)?
- Are the reference ("normal") ranges quoted in the study comparable with those in the situation of concern?
- Are the action limits (if relevant) quoted in the study appropriate to the situation with which you're concerned?

I: Is the new analytical test method well described and correctly validated?

- Has the accuracy of the new test method been validated?
- Has the precision of the new test method been validated?
- Are the analytical performance characteristics of the new test method (e.g., its accuracy, precision, and the diagnostic accuracy performance characteristics) comparable with the comparator method—and appropriate?
- Is there any evidence that the analytical performance of the new test method (i.e., accuracy and precision) has any impact on the health outcome (e.g., on the nature of the clinical decisions that will be made)?
- Do the problems addressed in the study match those posed by your question, or that of the inquirer?

C: Is the comparator test method well described and correctly validated?

- Has the accuracy of the comparator test method been validated?
- Has the precision of the comparator test method been validated?
- Are the diagnostic accuracy performance characteristics of the comparator method well described—either in the paper, or in referenced literature (e.g., is there a recognized "gold standard")?
- Is there any evidence that the analytical performance of the comparator test method (i.e., its accuracy and precision) has any impact on the health outcome (e.g., on the nature of the clinical decisions that will be made)?

> Remember that not all studies will necessarily have a comparator group, e.g., cohort studies in prognostic studies.

Change management: What changes will be needed to gain the benefit?

- Is there a clear vision of the benefits that will accrue from using the test in the way described in the study (i.e., what is the value proposition)?
- What changes may have to be made to the process of care? E.g., consider
  - Change in diagnostic tests?
  - Change in operational aspects of delivery of test?
  - Change in treatment protocol?
  - Change in monitoring the patient?
- What are the staff training and accreditation issues for the health professionals involved?
- Are there any risks for the patient?
- Are there any operational implications for the patient?
- How will the change be explained to the patient?
- What is the patient's view on the proposed change to practice?
- Is there an increase in financial expenditure involved with using the new test, and a saving to be made elsewhere in the organization(s) providing the package of care, or for the patient(s)?
- Who are the key personnel responsible for the departments and clinical groups involved in the change to the process of care?

> Remember that when applying tests, some change in practice will always be needed—at a minimum, interpreting the test result, making some sort of decision, and taking action—even if the action is "no action." In some circumstances there may be significant operational changes, e.g., when using POCT.

- Are the changes identified deliverable?
- Will it be possible to reallocate resources in order to make the necessary operational changes to the process of care and deliver the benefits?
- What is the expected time to deliver the change and is there an implementation plan?

O: Are the outcome measures realistic and robust?

- Are the outcome measures specifically stated and relevant?
- Is the time between testing and outcome assessment appropriate?
- Are the outcome measures described valid for this type of study application?
- Are the outcome measures used in the study applicable to the question being asked in the situation you are dealing with at the moment?
- Are the outcome measures used in the study assessed in the same way that you are considering? For example, will the length-of-stay identified in the study be applicable to your situation, and can the benefits be realized?

Remember, it can be helpful when developing your structured question to use the variations in the PICO formula, such as adding an "S" for "setting," "T" for "time," and "C" for "change management."

The links between and among these questions and the daily practice of laboratory medicine are shown below.

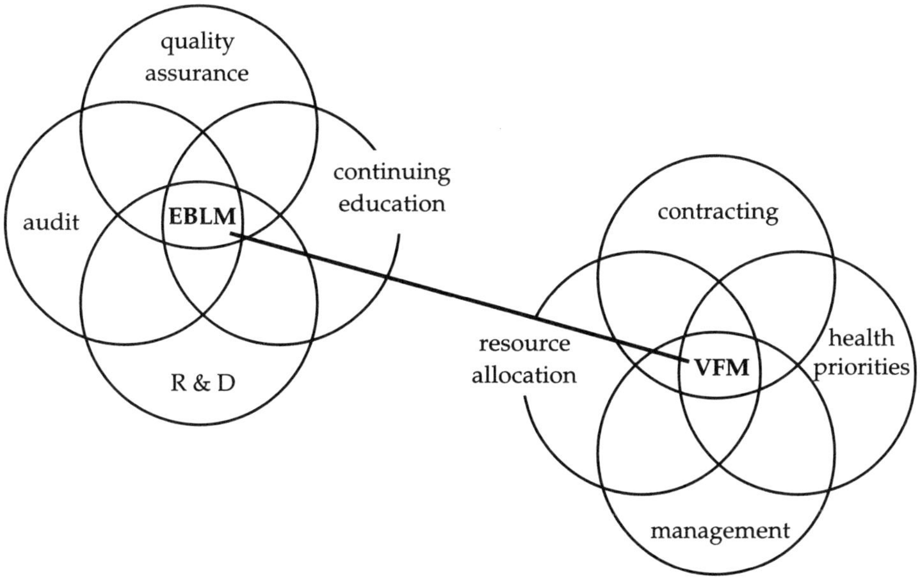

The key activities in laboratory medicine required to deliver quality and value-for-money (VFM)
Reprinted with permission from Price CP. Evidence-based laboratory medicine: supporting decision-making. Clin Chem 2000;46:1041–50.

Pause and Reflect

Ideally, you've been applying your own experience to the cases presented in this workbook, and to cases that have come up in your own setting. How have you managed? We suggest you assess your progress with a couple of cases of your own, and the questions that you asked when reviewing the evidence you used to help resolve a problem.

Case A Scenario. ....

....

....

....

....

P: ....

....

....

....

I: ....

....

....

....

C: ....

....

....

....

C: ....

....

....

....

O: ....

....

....

....

Note: We have included "C" for "change management" at this point, to cover the possibility that you are looking at evidence that will change practice. If you are simply responding to an inquiry, then the extra "C" may not be required. However, if you are considering introducing a new test or modality of testing, then you will want to include "C" to ensure that the change management issues are addressed.

Pause and Reflect

Case B Scenario.

P:

I:

C:

C:

O:

Continued

Pause and Reflect (Cont'd)

Now assess your competence and understanding in deriving the questions that are relevant to the problems you are dealing with in your day-to-day practice, using a scale of 1 (poor) to 10 (excellent), and note any particular issues that you find difficult to deal with.

P: ....

I: ....

C: ....

C: ....

O: ....

Issues to resolve: ....

What's your plan for resolving these issues?

Sample Applications to Practice

Let's walk through two clinical scenarios, to see how the evidence you've uncovered in your research can be applied to practice.

Clinical Scenario 1

Introducing the Use of BNP for the Management of Patients with Heart Failure

A cardiologist visits the laboratory having heard about a test for natriuretic peptides, and asks if it can be used in the management of heart failure. He explains some of the difficulties in managing patients with heart failure, in particular the need for a sensitive tool for the assessment of ventricular function. He thinks that the natriuretic peptide test may be a valuable addition to his monitoring armamentarium and asks the clinical chemist to consider making the test available for his clinic. The biochemist conducts a literature search and finds the paper published by Jourdain et al. *(4)*.

P: Is the patient (or population) similar to that described in the study?

- *Does the patient (or population) with whom you are now concerned match those described in the study?* The paper describes a study involving patients with heart failure with New York Heart Association scores II and III.
- *Are the patients (or population) featured in the study so different from those with whom you are concerned that the study results are not applicable to your population or patient?* The data may not be applicable in newly diagnosed disease with different severity.
- *Is the setting of the study comparable to the setting in question (e.g., primary or secondary care)?* A secondary care, ambulatory clinic setting was used. However, only stabilized HF patients were included in the study, so caution is advised in the application to your cardiologist's patients.
- *Are the reference ("normal") ranges quoted in the study comparable with those in the situation of concern?* Yes, we plan to use the same analytical method. However, one target BNP value of 100 pg/mL was used to guide management for stable patients included in the study.
- *Are the action limits (if relevant) quoted in the study appropriate to the situation with which you're concerned?* Yes, in part, because we plan

Note: This is an example in which use of "S" for "setting" can be helpful because the study is concerned with a secondary care clinic, while your question may be concerned with a primary care setting.

to use the same analytical method. However, the action limit (goal BNP level) of 100 pg/mL in this paper is a diagnostic cutoff derived from acute decompensated HF patients; this is obviously a very different population and purpose. This goal BNP level in newly diagnosed patients may not be applicable, or only with extra care, in the monitoring of these patients.

I: Is the new analytical test method well described and correctly validated?

- *Has the accuracy of the new test method been validated?* Yes.
- *Has the precision of the new test method been validated?* Yes.
- *Are the analytical performance characteristics of the new test method (e.g., accuracy, precision, and the diagnostic accuracy performance characteristics) comparable with the comparator method—and appropriate?* Not applicable in this scenario because comparison is being made with the current standard of care, which does not involve a diagnostic test.
- *Is there any evidence that the analytical performance of the new test method (i.e., accuracy and precision) has any impact on the health outcome (e.g., on the nature of the clinical decisions that will be made)?* Not known from reading this paper.
- *Do the problems addressed in the study match those posed by your question, or that of the inquirer?* Yes, in part, but with the caveat that the patients must be diligently stabilized, as in this study.

> Remember that clinicians may use signs and symptoms, or patient characteristics, e.g., weight for monitoring–and this can be considered a "test."

C: Is the comparator test method well described and correctly validated?

- *Has the accuracy of the comparator test method been validated?* It is currently the standard of care, which does not involve the use of a diagnostic test.
- *Has the precision of the comparator test method been validated?* Not applicable in this scenario.
- *Are the diagnostic accuracy performance characteristics of the comparator method well described—either in the paper, or in referenced literature (e.g., is there a recognized "gold standard")?* Current standard of care is well described, although it does include a number of subjective measures and may not be considered a "gold standard method."
- *Is there any evidence that the analytical performance of the comparator test method (i.e., its accuracy and precision) has any impact on the health outcome (e.g., on the nature of the clinical decisions that will be made)?* Not relevant in this scenario.

> It is important to read the study methodology very carefully. In this particular study, the therapy for all the patients was optimized over several months before the study of BNP for monitoring began. This represents an unusual patient population, and, as a result, the main criticism of this study is that the spectrum of patients included was very select. Consequently, it may not be representative of the patient group you are considering.

Change management: What changes will need to be made to gain the benefit?

- *Is there a clear vision of the benefits that will accrue from using the test in the way described in the study (i.e., what is the value proposition)?* Yes, reduction in cardiac events; improved morbidity and mortality, provided the patient spectrum is the same.
- *What changes may have to be made to the process of care? e.g., consider*
  - *Change in diagnostic tests?* Use of a test at the time of the clinic visit.
  - *Change in operational aspects of delivery of test?* Use of a point-of-care test.
  - *Change in treatment protocol?* More frequent treatment changes were made on the basis of the natriuretic peptide measurement in the study.
  - *Change in monitoring the patient?* Yes, as in the above and with additional care in newly diagnosed patients.
- *What are the staff training and accreditation issues for the health professionals involved?* For clinicians, interpretation of natriuretic peptide results; for nurses, the use of the POCT system and quality control of measurements, etc.
- *Are there any risks for the patient?* Those associated with poor training in the use of test to guide clinical decision making and in the use of the POCT system itself. The strategy would not be appropriate for newly diagnosed patients, as the evidence supplied was obtained in patients who had been carefully stabilized.
- *Are there any operational implications for the patient?* The patient will have a test during the clinic visit but may expect to have fewer clinic visits overall, and also better health outcomes (e.g., fewer hospital admissions). It may be necessary to redesign the patient flow in the clinic.
- *How will the change be explained to the patient?* By clinician at first clinic visit and when the test result is received.
- *What is the patient's view on the proposed change in practice?* It is likely to be positive; an early poll of patients about the intended change was very positive.
- *Is there an increase in financial expenditure involved with using the new test, and a saving to be made elsewhere in the organization(s) providing the package of care, or for the patient(s)?* There will be the

additional cost of the test, but there will be downstream savings through reduced utilization of other health resources, (e.g., fewer clinic visits, fewer hospital admissions).

- *Who are the key personnel responsible for the departments and clinical groups involved in the change to the process of care?* Cardiologists, nursing staff, pharmacists, laboratory staff (for oversight of quality control), and hospital managers.
- *Are the changes identified deliverable?* Yes.
- *Will it be possible to reallocate resources in order to make the necessary operational changes to the process of care and deliver the benefits?* Yes.
- *What is the expected time to deliver the change and is there an implementation plan?* Eight months for complete implementation, with an audit of progress every two months up to six months, and then once every six months after the start of the service and completion of implementation phase.

O: Are the outcome measures realistic and robust?

- *Are the outcome measures described valid for this type of study application?* Yes.
- *Are the outcome measures used in the study applicable to the question being asked in the situation you are dealing with at the moment?* Yes.
- *Are the outcome measures used in the study assessed in the same way that you are considering? For example, will the length-of-stay identified in the study be applicable to your situation, and can the benefits be realized?* Yes.

Clinical Scenario 2

Introducing *Chlamydia* Screening Using a PCR Method

The head of the Obstetrics and Gynecology Department has approached you to discuss the introduction of screening for *Chlamydia trachomatis* in the family planning clinic using a DNA-based detection method. She points out a study in which this approach has been compared with no screening, and with screening based on an immunoassay-based method *(5)*. You undertake a quick literature search and find a number of papers investigating the use of DNA-based methods for screening in a number of populations, and also a systematic review *(6)* that concludes that DNA-based methods offer the benefits of higher detection rates. You decide to proceed with your business case based on the paper identified at the outset as it most closely reflects the needs of the inquirer.

P: Is the patient (or population) similar to that described in the study?

- *Does the patient (or population) with whom you are now concerned match those described in the study?* The study was conducted in a family planning clinic setting, which matches that of the inquirer. Furthermore, the authors in their modeling show that the economic benefits depend upon the prevalence of infection in the screened community—which are similar to those in the local community for which the screening program is being considered.
- *Are the patients (or population) featured in the study so different from those with whom you are concerned that the study results are not applicable to your population or patient?* The patient population is similar with the exception of being in another country. However, public health statistics suggest that the prevalence of the infection is similar in both settings.
- *Is the setting of the study comparable to the setting in question (e.g., primary or secondary care)?* Yes, with the proviso outlined above. Furthermore the current complication rates are similar to those in the study setting prior to the introduction of a screening program.
- *Are the reference ("normal") ranges quoted in the study comparable with those in the situation of concern?* It would be necessary to get experience with the chosen analytical method.
- *Are the action limits (if relevant) quoted in the study appropriate to the situation with which you're concerned?* It would be necessary to employ cut-off values obtained from local sites using the chosen assay and to consolidate experience from prospective analysis of local data.

I: Is the new analytical test method well described and correctly validated?

- *Has the accuracy of the new test method been validated?* Yes.
- *Has the precision of the new test method been validated?* Yes.
- *Are the analytical performance characteristics of the new test method (e.g., accuracy, precision, and the diagnostic accuracy performance*

characteristics) comparable with the comparator method—and appropriate? This scenario involves setting up a new service. However, there is an alternative method available based on immunoassay. The systematic review *(6)* concluded that the DNA-based tests offered better sensitivity of detection.

- *Is there any evidence that the analytical performance of the new test method (i.e., its accuracy and precision) has any impact on the health outcome (e.g., on the nature of the clinical decisions that will be made)?* DNA-based methods will detect more cases of infection compared with immunoassay methods.
- *Do the problems addressed in the study match those posed by your question, or that of the inquirer?* Yes.

C: Is the comparator test method well described and correctly validated?

- *Has the accuracy of comparator test method been validated?* The initial inquiry was about setting up a screening program, and so the comparator is "no screening." However the study points to a reduction in the complications of *Chlamydia* infection associated with the introduction of screening. Furthermore, DNA-based methods increase the rate of detection compared with immunoassay-based methods.
- *Has the precision of the comparator test method been validated?* Not applicable in this scenario.
- *Are the diagnostic accuracy performance characteristics of the comparator method well described—either in the paper, or in referenced literature (e.g., is there a recognized "gold standard")?* The incidence of the complications of *Chlamydia* infection—e.g., pelvic inflammatory disease, ectopic pregnancy, and infertility—in the study population are known, as well as the reduction in these rates associated with a screening program.
- *Is there any evidence that the analytical performance of the comparator test method (i.e., its accuracy and precision) has any impact on the health outcome (e.g., on the nature of the clinical decisions that will be made)?* Not relevant in this scenario.

Change management: What changes will need to be made to gain the benefit?

- *Is there a clear vision of the benefits that will accrue from using the test in the way described in the study (i.e., what is the value proposition)?* Yes, reduction in the incidence of ectopic pregnancies, pelvic inflammatory disease, and infertility.
- *What changes may have to be made to the process of care? E.g., consider*
  - *Change in diagnostic tests?* Introduction of a DNA-based test for *Chlamydia* in women attending family planning clinics.
  - *Change in operational aspects of delivery of test?* Patients invited to participate and samples sent to the laboratory for analysis.
  - *Change in treatment protocol?* Patients with positive results would be contacted to return to the clinic for treatment.
  - *Change in monitoring the patient?* Not necessarily relevant in this setting, although there are issues around patients who do not "attend" to receive the test result, which can have long-term consequences in the case of a patient who tests positive.
- *What are the staff training and accreditation issues for the health professionals involved?* For clinicians and nurses: explaining screening program, sample collection, explanation of results and treatment. For laboratory staff: performance of test and interpretation of results.
- *Are there any risks for the patient?* In addition to those of awareness of the impact of *Chlamydia* infection, understanding the importance of returning for treatment.
- *Are there any operational implications for the patient?* Specimen collection (cervical sampling preferred) and return for treatment.
- *How will the change be explained to the patient?* By clinician at first clinic visit and then at receipt of the test result.
- *What is the patient's view on the proposed change in practice?* An initial poll of patients indicated acceptance of the need for such testing. However, experience in this field has shown that a significant number of patients are lost-to-follow-up (i.e., they do not return for treatment). This is less likely to be an issue in a family planning context although this may still be an issue if the patients are recruited from primary care.

- *Is there an increase in financial expenditure involved with using the new test, and a saving to be made elsewhere in the organization(s) providing the package of care, or for the patient(s)?* Initial analysis suggests that in the local population the cost of providing the screening test will equate to about 12.5% (approximately $250,000) of the current cost of managing the complications (approximately $2,000,000). The investment in the laboratory will come from the savings made in hospital stay costs as a consequence of the reduction in complications associated with the infection.
- *Who are the key personnel responsible for the departments and clinical groups involved in the change to the process of care?* Clinicians and nursing staff from the Obstetrics and Gynecology Department, primary care physicians, laboratory personnel, and hospital managers.
- *Are the changes identified deliverable?* Yes.
- *Will it be possible to reallocate resources in order to make the necessary operational changes to the process of care and deliver the benefits?* The case is made on this assumption.
- *What is the expected time to deliver the change and is there an implementation plan?* Eighteen months for complete implementation, with an audit of progress at three-month intervals (every three months up to month 18 after starting the service), and then once every six months thereafter.

O: Are the outcome measures realistic and robust?

- *Are the outcome measures described valid for this type of study application?* Yes, a reduction in the complications associated with *Chlamydia* infection.
- *Are the outcome measures used in the study applicable to the question being asked in the situation you are dealing with at the moment?* Yes.
- *Are the outcome measures used in the study assessed in the same way that you are considering? For example, will the length-of-stay identified in the study be applicable to your situation, and can the benefits be realized?* Yes, the main outcome measures are clinical indices—namely the incidence of complications.

Now You Try It

Clinical Scenario 3

Now apply this process to your own case, using a question that you are concerned with answering in your own setting.

Make sure that you have done the following before you take this fourth step in the A5 cycle:

Describe the clinical scenario.

....

....

....

....

....

A1: Ask. Formulate your clinical question, using PICO. (Review pp. 49.)

P: ....

I: ....

C: ....

O: ....

Note: You can choose to include PICO variants "S" for "setting," "T" for "time," and "C" for "change management."

A2: Acquire. Find the evidence, using PubMed or another appropriate database. (Review "Overview: Steps in the Search Process," pp. 97.)

Type of question (diagnostic, therapy, prognostic, etc.):

....

Type of search (detailed systematic, systematic review, metaanalysis):

....

Database used: ....

Keywords/MESH terms: ....

....

Narrow results with Boolean terms or other features? ....

....

Relevant results: ....

....

....

....

....

....

A3: Appraise. Evaluate the evidence, using the appropriate checklist.
(See "Appraisal Checklists," pp. 126–127, and Appendix C, D, or E.)

Type of study: ....

Checklist used: ....

A4: Apply. Now work through the exercise below to apply the evidence to your clinical situation.

P: Is the patient (or population) similar to that described in the study?

- *Does the patient (or population) with whom you are now concerned match those described in the study? Important factors to consider: age, sex, ethnicity, stage in the evolution of the condition, severity of condition.* ....

  ....

- *Are the patients (or population) featured in the study so different from those with whom you are concerned that the study results are not applicable to your population or patient?* ....

  ....

- *Is the setting of the study comparable to the setting in question (e.g., primary or secondary care)?* ....

  ....

  ....

- *Are the reference ("normal") ranges quoted in the study comparable with those in the situation of concern?* ....

- *Are the action limits (if relevant) quoted in the study appropriate to the situation with which you're concerned?* ....

....

I: Is the new analytical test method well described and correctly validated?

- *Has the accuracy of the new test method been validated?* ....
- *Has the precision of the new test method been validated?* ....
- *Are the analytical performance characteristics of the new test method (e.g., accuracy, precision, and the diagnostic accuracy performance characteristics) comparable with the comparator method—and appropriate?* ....

....

- *Is there any evidence that the analytical performance of the new test method (i.e., its accuracy and precision) has any impact on the health outcome (e.g., on the nature of the clinical decisions that will be made)?* ....

....

....

- *Do the problems addressed in the study reported match those posed by the inquirer?* ....

C: Is the comparator test method well described and correctly validated?

- *Has the accuracy of comparator test method been validated?* ....
- *Has the precision of the comparator test method been validated?*

....

- *Are the diagnostic accuracy performance characteristics of the comparator method well described—either in the paper, or in referenced literature (e.g., is there a recognized "gold standard")?*

....

- *Is there any evidence that the analytical performance of the comparator test method (i.e., its accuracy and precision) has any impact on the health outcome (e.g., on the nature of the clinical decisions that will be made)?* ....

....

Change management: What changes will need to be made to gain the benefit?

- *Is there a clear vision of the benefits that will accrue from using the test in the way described in the study (i.e., what is the value proposition)?*

  ....

  ....

- *What changes may have to be made to the process of care? e.g., consider*

  - Change in diagnostic tests? ....

  ....

  - Change in operational aspects of delivery of test? ....

  ....

  - Change in treatment protocol? ....

  ....

  - Change in monitoring the patient? ....

  ....

- *What are the staff training and accreditation issues for the health professionals involved?* ....

  ....

- *Are there any risks for the patient?* ....

  ....

- *Are there any operational implications for the patient?* ....

  ....

- *How will the change be explained to the patient?* ....

  ....

- *What is the patient's view on the proposed change in practice?*

  ....

- *Is there an increase in financial expenditure involved with use of the new test, and a saving to be made elsewhere in the organization(s) providing the package of care, or for the patient?*

....

....

- *Who are the key personnel responsible for the departments and clinical groups involved in the change to the process of care?*

....

....

- *Are the changes identified deliverable?* ....
- *Will it be possible to reallocate resources in order to make the necessary operational changes to the process of care and deliver the benefits?*

....

....

- *What is the expected time to deliver the change and is there an implementation plan?* ....

....

O: Are the outcome measures realistic and robust?

- *Are the outcome measures described valid for this type of study application?* ....

....

- *Are the outcome measures used in the study applicable to the question being asked in the situation you are dealing with at the moment?* ....

....

....

- *Are the outcome measures used in the study assessed in the same way that you are considering? For example, will the length-of-stay identified in the study be applicable to your situation, and can the benefits be realized?* ....

....

Taking Stock

So, what have you learned?

As a result of working through this section, you are likely to now understand...

- How bringing together the practices of question formulation (PICO), searching, and critical appraisal enables you to express your clinical problem in the form of a structured question, which in turn enables you to determine if there is any good-quality evidence to help answer the question.
- How employing the PICO format helps you to determine whether the evidence you have found is relevant to, and can be applied to, your clinical problem.
- That structuring these questions using the PICO process helps determine the relevance of the evidence and identify the key issues that may arise when implementing the solution to the problem identified at the outset.
- How this process helps you address the important challenges of implementation.
- And appreciate the need for an implementation plan

> Incidentally, if you are unable to find any evidence to help answer your question, then the question will provide you with the basis for designing a study to obtain the necessary data. The types of questions illustrated in this section on applying evidence will give you further insight into aspects of the study design. (See also Appendix A).

> Many of the questions around implementation can also be applied to efforts to control the demand for laboratory investigation (e.g., an audit), especially when faced with the prospect (and in the presence of robust evidence to support the case) of having to decline the provision of unnecessary tests.

Pause and Reflect

Now assess your competence and understanding of the questions that are relevant to the problems you are dealing with in your day-to-day practice when applying evidence, using a scale of 1 (poor) to 10 (excellent).

P: ....

I: ....

C: ....

C: ....

O: ....

Write down any issues that you feel are still remaining having gone through the case scenarios:

P: ....

....

....

I: ....

....

....

C: ....

....

....

C: ....

....

....

O: ....

....

....

Now look back at the concerns that you had before you started to go through the case studies (see Part 2, Step A1, page 52). What changes have you noticed in how you think about and address these issues?

....

....

....

Summary: Applying Evidence in Practice

You are now gaining practical experience with using EBLM in your day-to-day practice; this is excellent experience to share with colleagues. If you still have some concerns or unanswered questions, then contact a colleague for help, put the problem up on a mailbase or listserv, and see what others think about the problems you are finding.

Remember, first and always, to use the PICO approach!

All of this experience, as well as the learning experience itself, will be an excellent resource for mentoring less experienced colleagues. You may find that some of these experiences are worthy of publication in a peer-reviewed journal, or in a newsletter. It is well known that sharing good practice, which is what this experience is about, is woefully inadequate in healthcare systems.

You could also use your experience as the basis of a journal club, which is one of the most successful ways of disseminating information. Indeed, this approach to problem solving can also be used in clinical governance and performance management exercises, for example, when assessing the appropriate use of tests.

Recap: Key Concepts

- To apply evidence effectively when resolving a problem requires understanding the question properly, ensuring that there is good evidence to support the change, and being aware of the changes in practice that will be required to deliver a good solution.
- Any application of evidence must always culminate in this key question: Do patients undergoing the diagnostic test fare better than similar untested patients? There is little point in performing a test unless there is the potential for benefit—whether it be clinical, operational or economic. Remember, though, that junior doctors are likely to request more tests as they gain experience.
- A generic checklist can be a helpful starting point to applying evidence to your clinical situation (see Appendix G).

References

1. Price CP. Evidence-based laboratory medicine: supporting decision-making. Clin Chem 2000;46:1041–50.
2. Devillé WL, Buntinx F, Bouter LM, et al. Conducting systematic reviews of diagnostic studies: didactic guidelines. BMC Med Res Methodol 2002 Jul 3;2:9.
3. Sackett DL, Haynes RB. The architecture of diagnostic research. BMJ 2002;324:539–41.
4. Jourdain P, Jondeau G, Funck F, et al. Plasma brain natriuretic peptide-guided therapy to improve outcome in heart failure: the STARS-BNP Multicenter Study. J Am Coll Cardiol 2007;49:1733–9.
5. Howell MR, Quinn TC, Brathwaite W, et al. Screening women for *Chlamydia trachomatis* in family planning clinics: the cost-effectiveness of DNA amplification assays. Sex Transm Dis 1998;25:108–17.
6. Watson EJ, Templeton A, Russell I, et al. The accuracy and efficacy of screening tests for *Chlamydia trachomatis*: a systematic review. J Med Microbiol 2002;51:1021–31.

STEP A5: ASSESS—Audit the Process

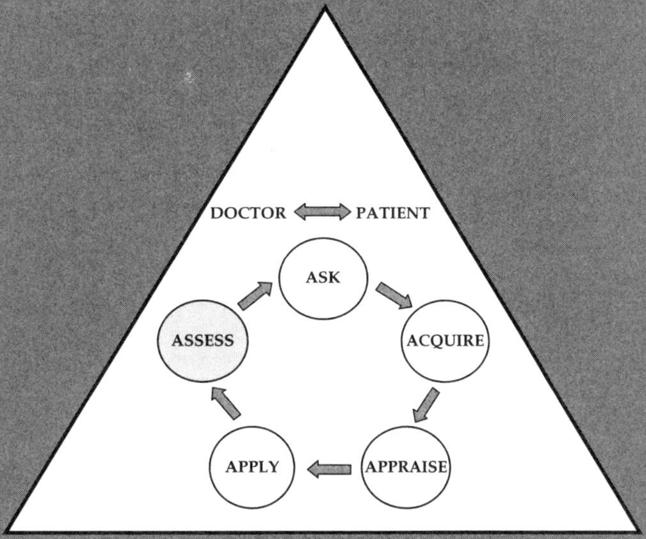

In this chapter

- Overview: EBLM as a process of lifelong learning
- Assimilating EBLM principles
- Assessing/auditing your performance
- Engaging in change management
- Taking stock: the audit process
- Summary: test yourself

Overview: EBLM As a Process of Lifelong Learning

The practice of Evidence-Based Medicine (EBM) has been described as a process of lifelong learning. The knowledge required to practice in any branch of medicine is such that it is likely you will regularly be challenged about your expertise in a particular situation.

> Remember in the definitions of Evidence-Based Medicine we referred to the process of lifelong learning. This is the final step in that process—checking that it works.

At the "big picture" level, the tapestry of healthcare is constantly changing with respect to demographics, including lifestyles and disease epidemiology, and expectations for, and financial pressures on, healthcare provision. Consequently, we constantly search for ways of responding to these changes.

At a more parochial level (in laboratory medicine, for example), new knowledge is constantly being synthesized, with new biomarkers developed, new applications for biomarkers demonstrated, and suggestions that established markers are becoming redundant. Knowledge management is therefore a dynamic process. The key is to be aware of this reality, know how to deal with it, and learn from it.

Applying the principles of the EBLM A5 cycle in your daily work ensures that you are indeed engaged in dynamic knowledge management—i.e., you are becoming a lifelong learner.

Key Concept

"Assess" in the A5 cycle means auditing (the effectiveness of) the EBLM process, and at this point looking at (i) how effectively you have picked up the skills described and illustrated in this book, and (ii) how effectively you are using these skills.

Some examples of the challenges that you may face and learn from are listed in the box below. Note that they are all phrased as questions!

Have You Encountered Any of These Questions?

- ❑ *What is the meaning of a serum bilirubin of 2.2. mg/dL (37 μmol/L) in an apparently healthy man who chose to have a "well-person screen"?*
- ❑ *How do I interpret an NT-proBNP result in a patient with chronic renal failure?*
- ❑ *What are the analytical performance specifications required for tests that are used in a Down syndrome screening program?*
- ❑ *Can measurement of natriuretic peptide help to guide therapy in patients with heart failure?*
- ❑ *Will the measurement of protein S100 help in the management of patients with melanoma?*
- ❑ *Should you provide an adiponectin testing service?*
- ❑ *Why have the requests for C-reactive protein risen by 75% over the last 18 months?*
- ❑ *Why do we measure lactate dehydrogenase?*
- ❑ *Why are your costs for providing ACTH measurements 20% higher than those of the laboratory 20 miles away?*
- ❑ *Will point-of-care testing for PT/INR monitoring in the community improve the health outcomes in patients on coumadin (warfarin) therapy?*
- ❑ *Could you provide a thyroptropin assay service for our one-stop thyroid clinic, and what would we have to change to make it work effectively?*
- ❑ *We want to be able to screen all patients for MRSA and* C difficile *prior to hospital admission for an elective procedure. What would you recommend?*
- ❑ *We have been working with our pharmacists on the issue of managing patients with diabetes in the community. What is the evidence on managing patients with diabetes in this setting?*

Pause and Reflect

In the box above, put a ✓ next to the problems you've dealt with, either as a result of working through the exercises in this book or encountering them in your practice. Then, reflecting on those items, score your responses to the following questions, using a scale of 1 (not at all or to a low degree) to 10 (very well or to a high degree).

- On average, how well/effectively can you deal with the problems listed? ....
- Were you able to learn something from dealing with these problems? ....
- How much has using the EBLM process changed your practice? ....
- Has using EBLM helped you to deal with other clinical issues that arose (i.e., was there a more generic benefit to use of the process)? ....

Notes for further study: ....

Assimilating EBLM Principles

The sample questions in the "Have You Encountered These Questions?" box (page 178) cover a wide area of practice including **analytical performance** of tests, **interpretation** of test results, **new applications** of a test, tests and their **impact on health outcomes**, the use of tests in **process change**, as well as **audit** in relation to **financial and clinical governance**. These are all the areas that can be addressed by applying the EBLM A5 cycle.

How are you assimilating the knowledge gained from learning about, and applying, the principles of EBLM?

Are You Using Your EBLM Skills Effectively?

- *Are you aware of the clinical questions arising in your daily practice?*
- *Have you been able to convert these questions into answerable questions, e.g., by using the PICO approach?*
- *Have you been able to perform searches to help you with your questions?*
- *Has critical appraisal been a helpful tool for you?*
- *Have you been able to apply the new knowledge (evidence) that you have gleaned?*

Remember, too, the PICO variants: "S" for "setting," "T" for "time," and "C" for "change management."

We suggest that you keep a record or journal of situations in which you have gained experience using the EBLM A5 cycle, together with the tips you have learned from applying these principles. These notes will not only be of value to you, but also to your colleagues, and provide a rich source of material when you are involved in training and continuing education activities. See the "Learning Log" on the next page.

Learning Log

We have included two examples from our own logs; you can add more.

Question	Skill Tip	Outcome
Does POCT for HbA1c lead to improved outcomes?	*Using the S for setting and C for change management helped in the critical appraisal of the paper by Cagliero et al., referred to in Part 2, Step A3, and in Appendix F, and the Khunti et al. paper referred to in Appendix F.*	*Identified possible reasons for the discrepancy between the findings of two studies.*
Will introduction of screening for Chlamydia *improve health outcomes?*	*Devising the PICOS questions can identify the research studies that need to be undertaken to support a a policy decision. (See the clinical scenario described in Part 2, Step A4, on pages 159–163, and the operational case study on page 78, and a suggested answer to that question on page 79.)*	*Identified the research agenda, business cases, and implementation strategy that might follow from a policy decision.*
....	....	....
....	....	....
....	....	....
....	....	....
....	....	....
....	....	....
....	....	....
....	....	....
....	....	....
....	....	....
....	....	....
....	....	....
....	....	....
....	....	....
....	....	....

Assessing/Auditing Your Performance

Now let's take a detailed look at each of the questions about using your EBLM skills effectively.

Are you aware of clinical questions arising in your daily practice? You're not doing your job properly if no questions that need answers are arising; clearly no health professional knows all the answers! When one of your colleagues has an unanswered question, how do you react?

- *When you receive an inquiry from a clinician do you think of it as being a question that you want to convert using the PICO approach?*
- *Do you consider other issues as potential PICO-applicable questions, e.g. complaints, requests for help?*
- *When you do not know or understand something, do you think about it as a question?*
- *How many times in a week do you respond to challenges by thinking of the questions being asked, or questions that you need to ask?*

Record some examples of issues that have arisen in your daily practice, where you have, or have not, thought about these issues in terms of the question(s) being asked as problems that can be investigated and then solved.

....

....

....

....

....

....

....

....

....

....

....

....

....

Have you been able to convert these questions into answerable questions, e.g., using the PICO approach? The PICO approach helps you think methodically about the issue as a problem that has a solution, and lays the groundwork for searching for the best evidence to answer the question.

- *Have you been successful in converting general questions into structured answerable questions?*
- *Have you been able to use the PICO approach consistently?*
- *Are there times when the PICO approach does not work?*
- *Does the PICO approach translate easily to the varying questions that present themselves to you?*
- *Are you able to identify your patient or population accurately and relate to the evidence that you find?*
- *Are you able to identify the outcomes that you are seeking when responding to an inquiry?*
- *Has constructing PICO questions become easier?*
- *Do you now find yourself using PICO in a widening range of situations when a query arises?*

We suggest that you record some examples of issues that have arisen in your daily practice, where you have been successful in translating the issue to an answerable question—and where you have encountered problems—or failed. In the latter case you might find it helpful to discuss the problem with a colleague.

....

....

....

....

....

....

....

....

....

....

....

Remember there are interpretations of the basic PICO formula. For example, "P" may stand for "patient" or "population," and "C" may not always be needed. Have you also used the PICO variants ("S" for "setting," "T" for "time," and "C" for "change management")?

Have you been able to perform searches to help you with your questions? Remember that the elements in the formulated question drive the search. The search itself may utilize a number of internet resources (see pages 95–96 for a listing). Of these, PubMed is the most useful source for searching in everyday practice, e.g., when receiving a telephone call, a visit from a clinician, or on ward rounds.

- *Have you found useful information when conducting searches?*
- *Have you learned or developed a technique that meets your needs and generates success on a regular basis?*
- *Do you use a structured approach or is it a bit "hit-and-miss"?*
- *Are you using MeSH terms?*
- *Have you used a range of resources? E.g., have you used PubMed and the Web of Science?*
- *Have you tried Google?*
- *Have you tried any of the resources listed in Part 3?*
- *Do you use the "related articles" feature of the database(s)?*
- *Do you use the "reviews" feature?*
- *Have you sought help with your search from a librarian?*
- *Have you compared your results from searching with those obtained by a librarian?*

We suggest that you record some examples of searches from questions that have arisen in your daily practice, where you have been successful in finding helpful papers—and where you have encountered problem—or failed to do so. In the latter case you might find it helpful to discuss the problem with a colleague.

....

....

....

....

....

....

....

....

Has critical appraisal been a helpful tool for you? Critical appraisal can be seen as "sorting the wheat from the chaff" and is the key to gaining experience in knowing when and how to apply what you learn to your clinical setting. Resources for critical appraisal can be found in Appendices C–E.

Speaking of critical appraisal, remember that you are assessing how well you are using the EBLM skills you have been acquiring AND how effective you are in using these skills.

- *Have you critically appraised any papers that have arisen from your searches?*
- *Do you feel this has helped discern better evidence?*
- *Have you become more familiar with the appropriate statistical approach to the treatment of data?*
- *Do you know what statistics are appropriate for the different study designs developed to respond to the questions being asked?*
- *Do you think this would enable you to offer a succinct critique of the evidence from a paper, which would impact the response you give to the initial inquirer?*
- *Has this process of critical appraisal helped you when reading papers that describe studies related to the application of diagnostic tests?*
- *Would this experience help you to design a study that would be able to provide robust evidence?*
- *Would this experience help you to contribute to the production of a guideline?*
- *Would this experience help you when reading and evaluating a guideline?*
- *Would this experience help you to write a paper on the application of a diagnostic test?*

We suggest that you record some examples of critical appraisals that have been conducted following questions that have arisen in your daily practice, situations in which you have been successful—and where you have encountered problems—or where you have failed. In the latter case you might find it helpful to discuss the problem with a colleague.

....

....

....

....

Have you been able to apply the new knowledge (evidence) that you have gleaned? Knowledge is not useful unless it can be applied; an unanswered question can be viewed as a failure in one's duty—even if the answer is a negative.

- *Using the steps outlined above, have you been able to provide answers to inquiries you've received?*
- *Are these answers more robust than before you used this approach—namely, were you able to formulate an answerable question, search the literature, and then find and critically appraise the evidence that was relevant to your inquiry?*
- *Do you feel your inquirers are more satisfied?*
- *Do you now find yourself using PICO "in your head" or do you have to "spell it out" in the conversation when a query arises?*
- *Does knowing the question expressed in PICO terms and the response help you to formulate a strategy for any change management that is required?*

Remember that one of the PICO variants is "C" for "change," and applying knowledge sometimes requires a change to the way things are done—and that it is only with this change that benefit is achieved.

We suggest that you record some examples where you have been able to apply Steps A1 to A4 of the EBLM cycle, following questions that have arisen in your daily practice. Where have you been successful—and where have you encountered problems—or failed to succeed? In the latter case you might find it helpful to discuss the problem with a colleague.

....

....

....

....

....

....

....

....

....

....

....

....

Engaging in Change Management

The steps of a change process can be described in this way:

- *Analyze current situation*
- *Develop shared vision of the future*
- *Sell vision to involve stakeholders and gain commitment*
- *Establish the implementation team and timetable*
- *Communicate constantly*
- *Persist and persevere*
- *Celebrate success*

Key Concept

> Invariably answering questions successfully requires change; successful application of the A5 cycle requires the engagement of change management.

We suggest that you record some examples where you have been able to apply a change management strategy to improve a process or outcome, as outlined above. Where have you been successful—and where have you encountered problems—or failed? In the latter case you might find it helpful to discuss the problem with a colleague.

....

....

....

....

....

....

....

....

....

....

....

....

Taking Stock: The Audit Process

Audit is a process of continuing evaluation and learning; along with assessment, it is an integral part of the A5 EBLM cycle.

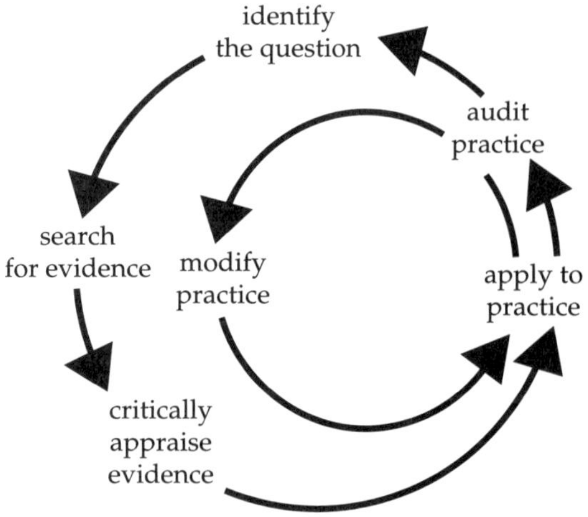

The place of audit in the EBLM cycle.

Reprinted with permission from Price CP. Evidence-based laboratory medicine: supporting decision-making. Clin Chem 2000;46:1041–50.

Barth (1) described the process of audit in "practical everyday terms":

- What you should be doing
- What you are doing
- Why are you not doing it?
- What you need to do to make it better
- Is there an improvement?

Collinson (2) has illustrated the role in which the audit process can be the starting point of good quality management, beginning with the question posed in Barth's list, and then leading into a search for evidence—and the EBLM A5 cycle. He also illustrated how an audit can then play an important role in initiating primary research, as well as (later in the process) the production of guidelines.

Key Concept

Audit is an important part of quality management in both laboratory and clinical practice. Audit is a crucial part of the EBLM cycle, and the components of the EBLM cycle feed the audit process. It follows, therefore, that the principles and practice of EBLM are central to good quality management and clinical practice.

Summary: Coming Full Circle

It is our hope that by using the principles of EBLM to work through the clinical examples in this workbook, you have become more proficient in applying the EBLM A5 cycle to questions that arise in your clinical setting. We also hope that you will pass on your knowledge to others through teaching and mentoring. In this way you ensure that you and your staff are indeed applying the best available scientific evidence to diagnostic challenges, and in the process, positioning the clinical laboratory to play a central role in patient care and clinical decision making.

See Appendix H—it offers an excellent opportunity to review key learning points presented in this workbook.

References

1. Barth JH. The role of clinical audit. In: Price CP, Christenson RH, eds. Evidence-Based Laboratory Medicine: From Principles to Outcomes. Washington, DC: AACC Press, 2003:209–24.
2. Collinson PO. The role of audit in laboratory medicine. In: Price CP, Christenson RH, eds. Evidence-Based Laboratory Medicine: Principles, Practice, and Outcomes, 2nd ed. Washington, DC: AACC Press, 2007:347–73.

Part 3

Additional Helpful Resources in the Practice of EBLM

In this chapter

- Glossary of commonly encountered terms
- Useful calculations and worked examples
- Useful resources: websites, sources of evidence, sources of guidelines
- Additional reading

Glossary of Commonly Encountered Terms*

AGREE (Appraisal of Guidelines for Research and Evaluation). A framework for assessing the quality of clinical practice guidelines. See later section for URL.

Attrition bias. Refers to systematic differences among the comparison groups in the loss of participants from a study and how they were accounted for in the results.

Audit. Process of evaluating the effect or impact of applying an evidence-based strategy. See also Step A5, "Clinical Audit," (pages 175–189).

Bayes' theorem. A formula that relates the conditional and marginal probabilities of stochastic (or random) events. In its simplest form it states that Post-test odds = Pre-test odds × likelihood ratio. See also later reference to the Fagan nomogram.

Before-and-after study. When one approach for use of a test is assessed in a defined population of patients for a defined period of time, then an alternative approach in a similar population (or the same population) is assessed. For example, a first group might be patients attending primary care with particular symptoms who would be studied for six months with a test from the main laboratory; the second group would have similar characteristics and be studied with POCT for the same analyte over the next six months. This is generally considered to be a better approach when adding on tests rather than when changing the test completely (1).

Bias. Observance of deviation of inferences or results (effects) from the true value. In EBLM the term "bias" is used when discussing the impact on study results. Bias can be due to (i) attrition, (ii) confirmation, (iii) differential verification, (iv) disease progression, (v) inappropriate reference test, (vi) incorporation, (vii) language, (viii) observer or operator, (ix) partial verification, (x) performance, (xi) publication, (xii) review, (xiii) selection, and/or (xiv) patient spectrum *(1)*.

---

*Every effort has been made to present clear and up-to-date definitions of the clinical terms, listed here, that are important with regard to their use in and application to EBLM. Sometimes we found it helpful to consult other resources for a precise, definitive explanation of the term. In such instances, references have been provided so that readers can consult these sources for more detail.

Blinding. A technique in experimental study design where either the caregiver who administers care to the patient or the patient (or both in the case of "double blinding") are unaware of the test result or treatment. Blinding helps to minimize the risk of results being influenced by the individuals undertaking the research. Examples where blinding is used include (i) the selection of patients entered into a trial, or a particular arm of a trial (as in a treatment trial); (ii) the establishment of the definitive diagnosis (as in a diagnostic accuracy study); or (iii) the reading of the test result using the reference method (as in a method comparison study).

Case-control study. In the case of a diagnostic test, a case-control study is a retrospective study in which you compare a cohort of patients with the same condition. One subset has the outcome of interest (the case) and the other does not have the outcome. Investigators can look at the distribution of the results in the two subsets of the populations to see if they are different. This study design would be used when investigating the prognostic value of a test. See Appendix A, "Appropriate Study Design."

CASP (Critical Appraisal Skills Programme). Offers a set of critical appraisal tools for evaluating a variety of study types, including diagnostic, economic, qualitative, randomized controlled trials, case control, and cohort studies, as well as systematic reviews.

CAT (Critically Appraised Topic). This is a way of summarizing evidence, which can then be stored for later use, e.g., in teaching.

Clinical audit. Systematic critical analysis of the quality of medical care, including the procedures for diagnosis and treatment, the use of resources and the resulting outcome and quality of life for the patient *(2)*. See Step A5, "ASSESS—Audit the Process," pages 175–189.

Clinical decision analysis. A formal method for reaching a decision. Healthcare professionals routinely complete this task many times each day, identifying possible options, inherent risks in each considered choice, and the odds of these risks occurring. Depending on the individual and the situation, the outcome variables may differ for different decisions, e.g., time, money, personal values and preferences, or satisfaction *(3, 4)*.

Clinical practice guideline. A group of systematically developed statements to assist and help guide practitioner and patient decisions about appropriate healthcare for specific clinical circumstances.

Cohort study. A "cohort" is a clearly identified group of people. A cohort study follows that group over time, and reports on what happens to them. A cohort study is an observational study, and it can be prospective (following people forward over time) or retrospective (looking at what happened in the past). See also Appendix A.

Comorbidity. The effect that all other diseases and conditions an individual patient might have, other than the primary disease of interest.

Confidence interval (CI). A means of quantifying the uncertainty of measurement. It is usually reported as the 95% CI, and represents the range of values within which we can be sure with 95% probability that the true value for the whole population lies *(3)*.

Confirmation bias. The tendency to seek evidence that confirms a hypothesis rather than data that enables the testing of an alternative hypothesis.

Confounder variable. A factor that might adversely influence the results of a study, e.g., the association between a test and a disorder, or between the use of a test and an outcome. Examples of potential confounders in the former might include age, sex, and ethnicity. Potential confounders in the latter might include the quality of information available to the clinician using the test.

Continuous variable. As applied to a test result, a continuous variable is one for which, within the limits of the variable ranges, a continuum of values is possible. Examples of continuous variables include red cell count, blood glucose, and serum total cholesterol.

Cost-benefit analysis. Assessing the value of a test based on determining the cost of the intervention, in this case a test, compared with the value of the benefit, with both being measured in the same terms, e.g., U.S. dollars *(3)*. This is sometimes viewed in terms of willingness to pay.

Cost-effectiveness analysis. Assessing the net cost of providing the test as well as the outcome or benefit gained. The outcomes are reported as a single unit of measurement *(3, 4)*.

Cost-minimization analysis. Assessing the cost of two alternatives, e.g., tests or ways of delivering tests, when the outcomes are equal. This is typically used when comparing two manufacturers' products, with the objective of finding the lowest cost provider *(3)*.

Cost-utility analysis. Assessing the net value of providing the test as well as the outcome or benefit gained. The outcomes are reported in terms of Quality Adjusted Life Years (QALYs) *(3, 4)*.

Cross-sectional study. A study in which a test (or observation) is performed in a population of patients at a single point in time and any outcome or characteristic is measured at the same time.

Dependent variable. The term *dependent* and *independent* variables refer to values that change in relationship to each other. The *dependent* variables are those that are observed to change in response to the *independent* variables.

Diagnostic accuracy study. Studies designed to assess the accuracy of a test of interest (often called the "index test") in making a diagnostic decision. Ideally, results of the index test are compared with a reference standard for the diagnosis. The patient cohort in whom the test is to be used and the clinical setting should also be defined.

Diagnostic odds ratio. The ratio of the positive likelihood ratio and the negative likelihood ratio. It is used to describe the diagnostic characteristics of the test as a single term. Calculated from [(True positive × True negative) / (False positive × False negative)]; see later worked example.

Dichotomous variable. A variable that categorizes data into two groups, e.g., present or absent, positive or negative, above the cut-off or below the cut-off.

Differential verification bias. This can occur when all patients in the study do not receive the same reference method. For example, if the reference method is tissue biopsy and some subjects with negative index test results are not subject to this "gold standard" and undergo a different reference test, then overestimation of test accuracy can occur.

Disease progression bias. This is related to the length of time between performance of the test under evaluation and confirmation by the reference method. A long time between index test performance and diagnosis confirmation with the reference method may introduce bias due to a change in disease status.

Evidence-based healthcare. Application of the principles of evidence-based medicine (EBM) to all those professions involved in the provision of healthcare, including those involved in policymaking and management.

Evidence-based medicine (EBM). The conscientious, explicit, and judicious use of current best evidence in making decisions about the care of individual patients. EBM has also been defined as the integration of best research evidence with clinical expertise and patient values. See Part 1, pages 4–7.

Evidence-based laboratory medicine (EBLM). The conscientious, explicit, and judicious use of current best evidence on laboratory tests in making decisions about the care of individual patients.

Exclusion criteria. These are the criteria used to determine when a potential subject can not be allowed to participate in a clinical trial. The most important criteria used to determine appropriateness for clinical trial participation include age, sex, pregnancy state, type and stage of a disease, treatment history, and other medical conditions.

External validity. The criteria for external validity provide an insight into the whether the study findings can be generalized to patients who were not in the study, and judge whether the test being evaluated has been assessed according to accepted standards. Such criteria include (i) spectrum of disease, (ii) setting, (iii) previous tests, (iv) duration of disease before diagnosis, (v) co-morbid conditions, (vi) demographics of study population, (vii) performance of index test, (viii) use of cut-off values, (ix) index test performance, and (x) cases lost to follow up.

Fixed effect model. This is a statistical model that stipulates that the units under analysis (people in a trial or study in a meta-analysis) are the ones of interest, and thus constitute the entire population of units. Only within-study variation is taken to influence the uncertainty of results (as reflected in the confidence interval) of a meta-analysis using a fixed effect model. Variation between the estimates of effect from each study (heterogeneity) does not affect the confidence interval in a fixed effect model *(4)*.

Hazard ratio. The weighted relative risk over the whole study population. This term is similar to the relative risk.

Heterogeneity. Variability among studies in a systematic review. It can be helpful to distinguish between different types of heterogeneity. Variability in the participants, interventions, and outcomes studied may be described as *clinical heterogeneity*, and variability in trial design and quality may be described as *methodological heterogeneity (4)*.

Inappropriate reference test bias. This can occur when the reference test does not represent the best available comparator. This typically leads to overestimation of specificity; the degree to which this occurs depends on the disease prevalence in the target condition.

Incidence. The number (often expressed as a proportion) of new cases of the target condition in the population at risk, over a defined period of time.

Inclusion criteria. Standards or criteria that must be met in order for a subject to participate in a clinical trial. Usually the following criteria are used to determine appropriateness for clinical trial participation: age, sex, pregnancy status, type and stage of disease, treatment history, and other medical conditions.

Incorporation bias. Potential for bias when the index test or information related to the index test is included in the diagnostic criteria. A good example is when a creatine kinase-MB (i.e., a biochemical cardiac marker) result is "incorporated" in making the diagnosis of myocardial infarction in a study to assess the diagnostic accuracy of a troponin test (i.e., another cardiac marker).

Index test. The test that is being investigated or evaluated.

Indexing bias. See "Publication bias."

Intention-to-treat analysis. A method of analysis for randomized clinical trials in which all patients assigned to one of the interventions (which may be test and treatment) are analyzed together, regardless of whether or not they completed or received that intervention, in order to preserve randomization *(3)*.

Internal validity criteria. Standards used to determine whether there is a risk of systematic error or bias in the results of a study due to the design. In diagnostic accuracy studies, these standards include (i) use of a valid reference standard, (ii) definition of cut-off point for a reference standard, (iii) blind measurement of index and reference test, (iv) avoidance of verification bias, (v) index test interpreted independently of all clinical information, and (vi) study design, i.e., prospective or retrospective.

Language bias. Studies and findings showing positive results are more likely to be published in English language journals, and are therefore more likely to be examined and cited in evidence subsequently published.

Likelihood ratio (see calculation below). Positive and negative likelihood ratios can be calculated. The positive likelihood ratio is the probability that a positive result for a given test would be found in a patient having the target condition compared with the likelihood that a positive result would be found in a patient without the target condition. Negative likelihood ratio is the probability of a negative result in patients who have the target condition compared with the probability of a negative result in a patient who does not have the condition.

Meta-analysis. A set of statistical techniques for combining similar information from a number of different studies including similar patients to derive an overall, more accurate estimate of a treatment effect or characteristics of a test.

Moses-type SROC curve. See "SROC."

n-of-1 trials. This generally applies to treatments, in which a patient receives an experimental treatment over a period of time and then switches to an alternative or placebo treatment. Ideally both the patient and the clinician are blinded to which treatment is being given, and the outcomes are monitored. Typically the treatment periods are alternated until patient and clinician conclude that one of the treatments is clearly different, or not different. These are sometimes known as crossover studies *(3, 4)*.

Negative likelihood ratio (see calculation below). An estimate of the probability of the presence of disease if the test result is negative. Mathematically, it is the probability of a negative result in patients who have the target condition divided by the probability of a negative result in patients who do not have the condition. Calculated from [(1 − Sensitivity) / Specificity]; see later worked example.

Negative predictive value (see calculation below). The probability that the patient does not have the condition if the test result is negative. Calculated from [True negative / (True negative + False negative)]; see later worked example.

Normal (result). A result that lies within the distribution of test data found in a population with no evidence of disease.

Number needed to harm (NNH). The number of patients who, if they received the experimental treatment, would result in one additional patient being harmed, compared with patients who receive the control treatment.

Number needed to treat (NNT). The number of patients who need to be treated to achieve one additional good outcome compared with patients who receive the control treatment.

Observational study. A study where data are collected during routine utilization, reflecting use of the test in routine practice. Such studies are very dependent on the data that are collected, both in terms of the actual metrics, as well as the completeness of collection.

Observer or operator bias. This may occur if the person reading or interpreting the test result is aware of any information about the patient or the result of other investigations—including the index or reference test result. This is sometimes called "test review bias."

Odds. A ratio of the number of people experiencing the event of interest compared to the number of people who do not experience the event of interest. See also reference *3*.

Odds ratio (OR). The ratio of the odds of having the target condition in the experimental group relative to the odds of having the target condition in the control group.

Outcome. The consequence of an intervention, or combinations of interventions, e.g., the use of a diagnostic test, and/or a treatment.

Partial verification bias. Some subjects with a negative index test result are not subject to the reference test. These patients will be assumed to be true negatives and the number of false positive results will be underestimated, leading to incorrect assessment of sensitivity and specificity.

Performance bias. It refers to systematic differences in the care, other than the intervention under investigation, provided to participants in the comparison groups. For example, in an outcome study investigating the use of a new test, or modality of testing, performance bias would be likely if the clinical care differed between the intervention and the comparator arms of the study.

PICO. The acronym that describes the core of formulating a structured question that underpins the steps of EBM and EBLM. The letters stand for **P**atient (or **P**opulation), **I**ntervention, **C**omparator (or **C**ontrol), and **O**utcome.

Positive likelihood ratio (see calculation below). An estimate of the probability of disease if the test is positive. Calculated from [Sensitivity / (1 − Specificity)]; see later worked example.

Positive predictive value (see calculation below). This is the probability that the patient has the condition when the test result is positive. Calculated from [True positive / (True positive + False positive)]; see later worked example.

Post-test odds (see calculation below). The odds that the patient has the target condition after the test information is used in the diagnostic process. See the definitions below for the exact relationship between pre-test and post-test odds and pre-test and post-test probabilities.

Post-test probability (see calculation below). The proportion of patients with the positive (abnormal) result who have the target condition.

Power calculation. Statistical power calculations provide a means of determining the sample sizes required to control for errors in hypothesis testing. See "StatPages.net" for further discussion. See also examples on pages 210–212, following the Fagan nomogram.

Pre-test odds. The odds that the patient has the target condition before the test has been performed, i.e., before the knowledge of the test result is available.

Pre-test probability (or prevalence). The proportion of people with the target condition in the population at risk.

Prevalence. The proportion of people within the population (the frequency) with the target condition. See also reference *4*.

Prognosis. A *prediction* of how a patient's *disease* will progress, which outcomes will occur, and whether there is chance of recovery.

Publication bias. The tendency for positive results to achieve publication, and in higher quality peer-reviewed literature. Other common forms are (i) when the results of a study are published on more than one occasion; this may include publication on an initial cohort of patients and a further publication when a larger group of subjects has been recruited, and (ii) when negative results are not reported, e.g., when a study shows that there is no benefit from using a particular test. This is also referred to as "indexing bias."

QUADAS (Quality Assessment of Diagnostic Accuracy in Systematic Reviews). A quality assessment tool intended for performing systematic reviews to assess the quality of primary studies of diagnostic accuracy. See later section for url.

RAMMbo. An acronym that describes a checklist for critically appraising studies. The letters stand for **R**ecruitment, **A**llocation or **A**djustment, **M**aintenance, **M**easurement, **b**linded, and **o**bjective.

Random effects model. This is a statistical model sometimes used in meta-analysis in which both within-study sampling error (variance) and between-studies variation are included in the assessment of the uncertainty (confidence interval) of the results of a meta-analysis. If there is significant heterogeneity among the results of the included studies, random effects models will give wider confidence intervals than fixed effect models *(4)*.

Randomization. A method for assigning patients to test or treatment groups that is by chance, akin to tossing a coin *(3, 4)*.

Randomized controlled trial. A study design in which participants are randomly allocated into an experimental group or a control group and observed over a period of time for the outcomes of interest *(3, 4)*.

Reference standard. A term that describes the most accurate assessment of the truth. Thus in the assessment of an analytical method it would be the closest to the true value, while in a diagnostic accuracy study it would be the best method available for making a diagnosis. It is sometimes called the "gold standard."

Relative benefit increase. The proportional increase in rates of good outcomes between experimental and control groups in a trial.

Relative risk. The ratio of the event rate in the group exposed to the experimental intervention compared with the event rate in the group exposed to the control intervention *(4)*.

Relative risk reduction. The proportional decrease in rates of bad outcomes between experimental and control groups in a trial *(4)*.

Review bias. When the investigator is not blinded to results of the index test or the reference test. This leads to overestimation of test accuracy, particularly if results are in any way subjective. See also "Observer bias."

Risk ratio (RR). The ratio of the risk in the treated group divided by the risk in the control group.

ROC. The receiver operating characteristic (ROC) curve represents the pattern of diagnostic sensitivities and specificities observed when the performance of a test is evaluated over a continuum of diagnostic thresholds. It is derived from signal detection theory, and is a graphical plot of the [sensitivity vs. (1 − specificity)] for a binary classifier system, as its discrimination threshold is varied. The ROC curve can also be represented equivalently by plotting the frequency of true positives (TPR = true positive rate) vs. the frequency of false positives (FPR = false positive rate). It is also known as a relative operating characteristic curve, because it is a comparison of two operating characteristics (TPR and FPR) as the criterion changes.

Selection bias. This type of bias may occur when only a specific population is selected, e.g., a certain age group, when the test is intended for a broader spectrum of patients. It can often happen if the reference test is undertaken first, and is thought to play a part in the patients subsequently chosen to receive the index test.

Sensitivity (diagnostic; see calculation below). It is the proportion of subjects with the target condition who have a positive test result. Calculated from [True positive / (True positive + False negative)]; see later worked example.

SnNout. An abbreviation used to describe when a test has a high sensitivity (**Sn**); then a negative result (**N**; e.g., the test result is within the normal range, within the reference interval, etc.) can help to "rule out" (**out**) the diagnosis or clinical decision informed by the use of the test *(3)*.

Specificity (diagnostic; see calculation below). It is the proportion of people without the target condition who have a negative test result. Calculated from [True negative / (True negative + False positive)]; see later worked example.

Spectrum bias. This can occur in the evaluation of the test in a population which is not representative of that for which the test will be used. Exaggeration of test accuracy can result, such as when the test is evaluated in patients with the disease of interest and in healthy patients, rather than all patients for whom the test would normally be considered.

SpPin. An abbreviation used to describe when a test has a high specificity (**Sp**); then a positive result (**P**; e.g., when the test result is outside the normal or reference interval) can help to "rule in" (**in**) the diagnosis or clinical decision informed by the use of the test *(3)*.

SROC. The Summary Receiver Operating Characteristic (ROC) curve describes the distribution of sensitivities and specificities observed when the performance of a test is evaluated in a meta-analysis of several studies. An example is shown and explained below.

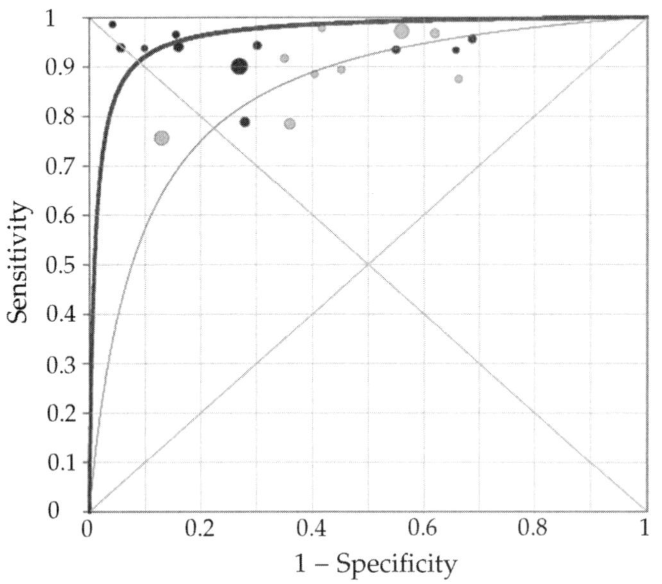

This shows the plots of true-positive rates versus false-positive rates from 22 studies of diagnostic accuracy of BNP testing for detection of heart failure (*5*, and abstracted from *6*). The results of the individual studies are plotted as circles, the areas of which are proportional to the number of individuals studied. The fitted lines represent Moses-type SROC curves. The two SROC curves shown are based upon studies using heart failure as the endpoint (dark circles with darker SROC curve) and those using LVSD as the endpoint (lighter circles with lighter SROC curve). A Moses-type SROC curve is based on summarizing the test accuracy of each study as a diagnostic odds ratio (DOR) and noting whether the DOR is related to the proportion of patients in the study having positive test results (which will change as a result of changes in the decision threshold), as explained in more detail in reference 6 and the original paper *(7)*. A summary of these techniques can be found in reference *8*.

STARD. An acronym for "**Sta**ndard for **R**eporting **D**iagnostic Accuracy;" describes the methodology for improving the quality of reporting of studies on diagnostic accuracy *(9, 10)*.

STEP. A program that describes how to explore the test performance characteristics of different screening and diagnostic tests. See later section for URL.

Systematic review. A summary of the literature that uses defined methods for performance of a systematic, comprehensive literature search and critical appraisal of the studies identified from the search. Appropriate statistical techniques are used to combine the data from valid studies. See also meta-analysis.

Target condition. A term used to denote the condition or disease that is being investigated, e.g., the use of natriuretic peptide measurement in the diagnosis of heart failure.

Validity. Also called logical truth, analytic truth, or necessary truth. The term "validity" as it occurs in logic refers generally to a property of particular statements and deductive arguments. Although validity and logical truth are synonymous concepts, the terms are used variously in different contexts *(11)*. Thus in terms of an analytical result in the clinical laboratory, validity refers to closeness to the true result. See also "Internal validity" and "External validity."

Useful Calculations

(taken from reference 6; modified with permission)

When using a test for making a diagnosis (or any decision), we will have populations of patients with the target condition and those without the condition. Each patient will have either a positive or negative result. In a dichotomous test, or variable, it is a simple positive/negative or present/absent decision. In the case of a continuous test, or variable, the conversion to a dichotomous variable is based on the use of a cut-off or decision point above or below which the individual patient result falls. The starting point in any calculations is a 2 × 2 contingency table.

	Disease present	Disease absent	Total
Test positive	TP	FP	TP + FP
Test negative	FN	TN	FN + TN
Total	TP + FN	FP + TN	TP + FP + FN + TN

Where: TP = true positive; FP = false positive; FN = false negative; TN = true negative

The diagnostic ***sensitivity*** of the test is provided by the number of true positive (TP) results divided by the total number of cases with confirmed presence of the disease [TP + false negative (FN)]: sensitivity = TP / (TP + FN).

The diagnostic ***specificity*** of the test is the number of true negative (TN) cases divided by the total number of cases with confirmed absence of the disease [TN + false positives (FP)]: specificity = TN / (TN + FP).

The ***positive predictive value (PPV or PV+)*** expresses the probability that a patient has a target disease, given that the test result is positive [TP / (TP + FP)].

The ***negative predictive value (NPV or PV−)*** expresses the probability that a patient does not have the target disease, given that the test result is negative [TN / (TN + FN)].

Though the sensitivity and specificity of a test may be high, the performance of the test as measured by the predictive value of a positive result may be poor (low PPV) when the disease prevalence is low in the population being tested. This dependence of PPV on disease prevalence has made it difficult to transfer results from evaluation studies directly into clinical practice, unless the prevalence in clinical practice will match that observed in the study.

The positive and negative ***likelihood ratios*** state how many-fold more likely particular test results are in patients with disease than in those without disease. For example, if the positive likelihood ratio is 10 for a test, then the probability of having a positive result in the diseased population is 10-fold the probability in the non-diseased population. This equates to using the test to "rule in" a diagnosis or decision. Likewise, if the negative likelihood ratio is 0.01, then the probability of having a negative result in the diseased population is one-hundredth that of having a negative result in the nondiseased population. This equates to using the test to "rule out" a diagnosis or decision. Thus, the farther a likelihood ratio deviates from unity (equal probabilities in the diseased and non-diseased populations), the more informative the test result corresponding to that likelihood ratio becomes. Negative likelihood ratios below 0.1 and positive likelihood ratios above 10 have been noted as providing convincing diagnostic evidence, whereas those below 0.2 or above 5 give strong diagnostic evidence *(12)*. However, these guidance figures will not apply when pre-test suspicions of disease are very high or very low. In these situations, more extreme negative and positive likelihood ratios will be needed to rule out and rule in diagnoses, respectively.

Considering the special case of a binary test in which the result may take on only two values—plus or minus—then likelihood ratios can be expressed in terms of sensitivity and specificity:

Positive likelihood ratio

$$L(+) = \frac{\text{Prob. positive result in patients with disease}}{\text{Prob. positive result in patient without disease}} = \frac{\text{Sensitivity}}{1 - \text{Specificity}}$$

Negative likelihood ratio

$$L(-) = \frac{\text{Prob. negative result in patients with disease}}{\text{Prob. negative result in patient without disease}} = \frac{1 - \text{Sensitivity}}{\text{Specificity}}$$

With use of Bayes' theorem, likelihood ratios can be directly applied to derive probabilistic statements regarding the likelihood of disease in an individual. The following formula is used:

$$\text{Post-test odds} = \text{pre-test odds} \times \text{likelihood ratio}$$

If the rate of heart failure in outpatients is 10 percent, and the likelihood ratio for a negative result is 0.15 as seen in the Craig et al. study *(5)*:

$$\text{Pre-test odds} = \text{prevalence} \;/\; (1 - \text{prevalence}) = 0.1 \;/\; 0.9 = 0.11$$

Applying Bayes' theorem to the pooled negative likelihood ratio:

$$\begin{aligned}\text{Post-test odds} &= \text{pre-test odds} \times \text{negative likelihood ratio}\\ &= 0.11 \times 0.15\\ &= 0.0165\end{aligned}$$

Converting post-test odds to post-test probability:

$$\begin{aligned}\text{Post-test probability} &= \text{post-test odds} \;/\; (1 + \text{post-test odds})\\ &= 0.0165 \;/\; (1 + 0.0165)\\ &= 0.016\end{aligned}$$

Thus, only about 2% of patients with a negative BNP result will have a diagnosis of heart failure. Calculations like this one are simplified by use of a Fagan pre-test/post-test probability nomogram (see below).

The ***diagnostic odds ratio (DOR)*** expresses the odds of positive test results in patients with disease compared with the odds of positive test results in those without disease [$L(+) / L(-) = (TP \times TN) / (FP \times FN)$]. Unlike the other statistics presented (sensitivity, specificity, and likelihood ratios), the diagnostic odds ratio summarizes the accuracy of a test as a single value, which makes it well-suited for use in meta-analysis. However, it may hide the fact as to whether the test is good for "rule in" or "rule out."

The Fagan nomogram

This is an example of the Fagan nomogram *(13)*, which can be used to determine the post-test probability. Starting with the pre-test probability value, draw a line through the likelihood ratio for the diagnostic test, continuing the line until it intersects the right-hand-most axis, which will provide the post-test probability. The line that has been drawn refers to the data described in the text on likelihood ratios.

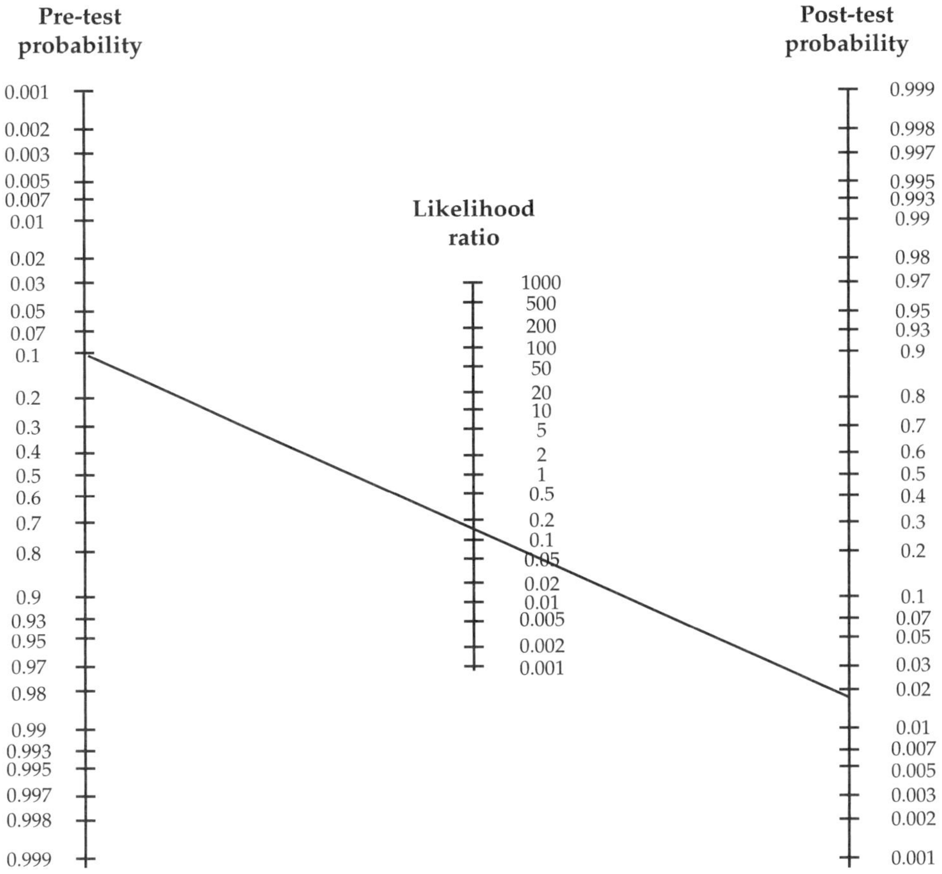

Power Calculation Examples

Diagnostic Performance: New Test for Detection of Prostate Cancer

Suppose you are in charge of new technology for an in vitro diagnostics company. An investigator contacts you claiming to have a new blood biomarker for prostate cancer screening in men with prostate-specific antigen (PSA) levels of <4 ng/mL. The investigator claims that the test is 93% sensitive for detecting men in this group who will have prostate cancer in the next five years. You know that in men over 50 years of age with a PSA value of <4 ng/mL the prevalence of prostate cancer is 20%, and that PSA is not sensitive for screening these individuals. Thus the new test is of potential interest to your company.

As part of due diligence, you need to verify the investigator's claim. You have access to an expensive sample bank from a screened cohort of men over 50, with 5-year disease outcomes. A large number have PSA <4 ng/mL. The PICOS question you formulate is as follows:

Patient	Men >50 years old with PSA <4 ng/mL diagnosed with prostate cancer
Indicator	Investigator's new test
Comparator	Men >50 years old with PSA <4 ng/mL with no prostate cancer
Outcome	Prostate cancer diagnosis within 5 years
Setting	Primary care screening in ostensibly healthy men

You wish to determine the number of cases and controls needed to help substantiate (or refute) the investigator's claim. As there is currently no screening test for the population, your view is that if the test can be shown to be close to 93%, then the test is potentially valuable. After some thought, you decide that a sensitivity that ranges down to 85% is reasonable. From the information you have, you wish to design the study such that if the sensitivity of cancer diagnosis is 93%, and you are willing to have a 8% uncertainty, i.e., you are willing to accept the claimed sensitivity of 93% if the test's diagnostic sensitivity can be demonstrated to be >85%. How large a sample size do you need to include in order to convincingly show, or disprove, that the sensitivity is 93% with an uncertainty of not more than 8% sensitivity?

A fundamental consideration of the sample size is to properly power your study. An appropriate sample size must be used to minimize what are termed type I and type II errors. To understand these errors it is first necessary to state the "null hypothesis." The null hypothesis in your problem is:

Null hypothesis: sensitivity of new test (p) = 93% (p0)

A type I error is the mistake of rejecting the null hypothesis, i.e., rejecting the test's claimed sensitivity, when in fact it is true. One way of viewing a type I error is that it is similar to a false negative result.

Type II error is the mistake of accepting the null hypothesis when it is false, i.e., accepting that the test is 93% sensitive when in fact it is not. One way of viewing a type II error is that it is similar to a false positive result. For evaluation of type II error, you must define a value, deemed not equivalent to the claimed 93% sensitivity, that you are unwilling to accept; here you have stated the test's sensitivity cannot be ≤85%. This sensitivity value is termed the "alternative hypothesis" and is defined for this example as follows:

Alternative hypothesis: sensitivity (p) ≤85% (p1, p1 < p0)

For dealing with type I error, you must specify an error rate at which you are willing to reject the null hypothesis while accepting the associated probability that the null hypothesis is in fact true. This error rate is termed "α," and by convention is set at a value 0.05, because this error rate for a type I error is generally accepted as being sufficiently small. On the other hand, the ability to reject the null hypothesis when it is false is termed power. Higher power also means smaller chance of making a type II error. Therefore, you must also specify a value for a type II error (β) that you are willing to accept, which is usually expressed as power, i.e., the probability of not committing a type II error (1−β). By convention a power of 0.8 is considered sufficient.

As stated above, by convention, the type I error rate is set at 0.05 and the study should be powered at 0.80; i.e., when the null hypothesis is rejected, the chance of it being true is only 0.05 or less while the chance of the alternative hypothesis being true is 0.2 or greater and, conversely, when the null hypothesis is accepted according to the test the chance of it being true is greater than 0.05 while the chance of the alternative hypothesis being true is less than 0.2. For a statistical test to achieve such an error rate and power the study must include enough subjects so that when it is completed there is at least 80% (4:1) chance that the null hypothesis of sensitivity being 93% will be rejected if the sensitivity is indeed 85% or less.

To see how many patients with specified characteristics must be recruited so that the study will have the specified significance level and power for its statistical test, you can use the calculator on the following website: http://stat.ubc.ca/~rollin/stats/ssize/b1.html

Alternatively, there are tables listed in many texts on statistics that provide similar information (for example: *Statistical Methods for Rates and Proportions* by Joseph L. Fleiss (2nd ed., 1981, John Wiley & Sons, NY), chapter 3.

Q: What is the total number of patients that must be recruited for a prospective cohort study given the prevalence of 20%?

A: For a power of 0.80 and a significance level of 0.05, you determine that you must have 44 subjects diagnosed with prostate cancer in the five years after testing. Because the prevalence of prostate cancer is 20% in the cohort, 220 total subjects (44 cases plus 176 non-diseased subjects) from the cohort must be included.

Outcome Study: POCT for HbA1c in the Community

This is based on the study reported by Khunti et al., who investigated the potential use of POCT for HbA1c in the management of type 2 diabetics in a primary care setting (14). The goal of their study was to increase the proportion of patients with "good glycemic control" from 40% (first group population proportion—i.e., the current state-of-play or current standard-of-care) to 50% (second group population proportion—i.e., sought after using POCT). They stipulated a significance of 5% (significance level 0.05 [α]) and a power of 80% ($1-\beta$, chance of detecting 0.8).

After completing a search on Google using "Sample size AND power calculations" the investigators used the power calculator referenced on "Power and Sample Size Programs" (http://www.biostat.ucsf.edu/sampsize.html#proportions), which is accessed by clicking on "Proportion Difference Power/Sample Size Calculation" (http://statpages.org/proppowr.html). This calculator is designed to "compute the sample size required to detect a difference between two proportions." The number required in each group (i.e., the conventional testing group [control] and the POCT group [intervention]) is 407. The authors decided they needed 400 in each group.

Note: These power calculation examples were developed with the assistance of Show-Hong Duh, Ph.D., University of Maryland School of Medicine, Baltimore, MD.

Useful Online Resources

Websites/URLs

http:www.jr2.ox.ac.uk/bandolier/band27/b27-2.html
An article from *Bandolier* entitled, "How Good is that Test?" *Bandolier* is a monthly newsletter about evidence-based healthcare, and is a very good source for such information on the net.

http://acb.rsmjournals.com/cgi/content/abstract/44/2/111
(Short-term access to a pdf of the full article is available for a fee.)
Review article in *Annals of Clinical Biochemistry*. Christenson RH; Committee on Evidence Based Laboratory Medicine of the International Federation for Clinical Chemistry Laboratory Medicine. Evidence-based laboratory medicine—a guide for critical evaluation of in vitro laboratory testing. Ann Clin Biochem 2007;44:111–30.

http://pubmedcentral.gov/articlerender.fcgi?artid=305345
Review article in *BMC Medical Research Methodology*. Whiting P, Rutjes AWS, Reitsma JB, et al. The development of QUADAS: a tool for the quality assessment of studies of diagnostic accuracy included in systematic reviews. BMC Med Res Methodol 2003;3:25.

http://www.bmj.com/cgi/content/full/324/7335/477
Review article in *BMJ*. Knottnerus JA, van Weel C, Muris JW. Evaluation of diagnostic procedures. BMJ 2002;324:477–80.

http://www.bmj.com/cgi/content/full/312/7023/71
Review article in *BMJ*. Sackett DL, Rosenberg WM, Gray JA, et al. Evidence based medicine: what it is and what it isn't. BMJ 1996;312:71–2.

http://www.bmj.com/cgi/content/full/317/7154/339
Review article in *BMJ*. Straus SE, Sackett DL. Using research findings in clinical practice. BMJ 1998;317:339–42.

http://www.pubmedcentral.nih.gov/articlerender.fcgi?tool=pubmed&pubmedid=16278748
Review article in *The Clinical Biochemist Reviews*. Hawkins RC. The evidence based medicine approach to diagnostic testing: practicalities and limitations. Clin Biochem Rev 2005;26:7–18.

http://www.clinchem.org/cgi/reprint/46/8/1041.pdf
Review article in *Clinical Chemistry*. Price CP. Evidence-based laboratory medicine: supporting decision-making. Clin Chem 2000;46:1041–50.

http://www.clinchem.org/cgi/reprint/47/8/1536
Review article in *Clinical Chemistry.* McQueen MJ. Overview of evidence-based medicine: challenges for evidence-based laboratory medicine. Clin Chem 2001;47:1536–46.

http://www.clinchem.org/cgi/reprint/50/5/806
Review article in *Clinical Chemistry*. Oosterhuis WP, Bruns DE, Watine J, et al. Evidence-based guidelines in laboratory medicine: principles and methods. Clin Chem 2004;50:806–18.

http://www.aacc.org/resourcecenters/resource_topics/ebm/Pages/default.aspx
American Association for Clinical Chemistry EBM resource, with links to other EBM and EBLM sites, as well as publications.

http://www.ifcc.org/index.php?option=com_content&task=blogcategory&id=64&Itemid=112
International Federation of Clinical Chemistry's Committee on Evidence-based Laboratory Medicine, with links to other EBLM sites, as well as educational materials and information on systematic reviews of diagnostic tests.

http://www.g-i-n.net/download/files/b33_davies.pdf
Davies P, Fitzgerald A, Alderson P. Feasibility of the QUADAS tool for quality assessment of diagnostic studies in guideline development. London: NHS National Institute for Health and Clinical Excellence (NICE), 2007.
Describes experience using the QUADAS tool and, in particular, looks at inter-rater reliability.

http://www.nice.org.uk/niceMedia/pdf/TAP_Methods.pdf
NICE. Guide to the Methods of Technology Appraisal. London: NHS National Institute for Clinical Excellence (NICE), 2004:47pp.

http://www.phru.nhs.uk/Pages/PHD/resources.htm
Site for the Public Health Resource Unit (PHRU), a not-for-profit National Health Service public health consultancy in the United Kingdom. Since 1997 PHRU has been working to promote health improvement and public health change and development. PHRU developed the Critical Appraisal Skills Programme (CASP), providing appraisal tools to evaluate a variety of study types including diagnostic, economic, qualitative, case control, and cohort studies, randomized clinical trials, and systematic reviews.

http://www.agreecollaboration.org/
Site for the AGREE (Appraisal of Guidelines for Research and Evaluation) Collaboration. The AGREE instrument is intended to provide a framework for assessing the quality of clinical practice guidelines. It was developed through discussion among researchers who have extensive experience and knowledge of clinical guidelines.

http://www.health.usyd.edu.au/step/
This site describes the objectives of a research program that seeks to explore the test performance characteristics of different screening and diagnostic tests. It is part of a wider public health program with an objective of understanding "which screening programs are worthwhile" and examining "how those that are worthwhile should be best implemented." The publications section of the website includes a list of peer-reviewed papers that report on the output from the program.

http://www.cebm.net/?o=1013
The site describes the work of the Centre for Evidence-Based Medicine (CEBM), "which was established in Oxford as the first of several centres whose broad aim is to promote evidence-based health care and provide support and resources." The site includes a number of critical appraisal forms, and also provides some very useful definitions and calculators, as well as lists of other EBM sites.

http://www.cebm.net/index.aspx?o=1216
Part of the CEBM site that describes the CATmaker, a software tool that "helps you create Critically Appraised Topics, or CATs, for the key articles you encounter about therapy, diagnosis, prognosis, [etiology]/harm, and systematic reviews of therapy."

http://www.cche.net/usersguides/main.asp
The Centre for Health Evidence (CHE) "is a multi-disciplinary initiative that brings universities, health organizations, and professional associations together. CHE supports the learning, teaching, and practice of evidence-based healthcare." CHE offers a variety of materials and check sheets including useful examples.

http://www.stard-statement.org/
Site describing the STARD initiative—toward complete and accurate reporting of studies of diagnostic accuracy—that has been reported in a number of journals.

http://www.shef.ac.uk/scharr/ir/netting/
A ScHARR Introduction to Evidence Based Practice on the Internet.

http://www.ahrq.gov/
Site for the Agency for Healthcare Research and Quality (AHRQ). The AHRQ is described as "the health services research arm of the U.S. Department of Health and Human Services (HHS), complementing the biomedical research mission of its sister agency, the National Institutes of Health." AHRQ is the umbrella organization for a number of research centers that "specialize in major areas of health care research [such as] quality improvement and patient safety, outcomes and effectiveness of care, clinical practice and technology assessment, and health care organization and delivery systems." Importantly, it is also "a major source of funding and technical assistance for health services research and research training at leading U.S. universities and other institutions" as well as a "science partner, working with the public and private sectors to build the knowledge base for what works—and does not work—in health and health care and to translate this knowledge into everyday practice and policymaking." It created the Effective Health Care initiative, and as part of that conducts Technology Assessments and Comparative Effectiveness Reviews.

http://www3.interscience.wiley.com/cgi-bin/mrwhome/106568753/HOME?SRETRY=0
Site for the Cochrane Library, which "contains high-quality, independent evidence to inform healthcare decision-making. It includes reliable evidence from Cochrane and other systematic reviews, clinical trials, and more."

http://www.crd.york.ac.uk/crdweb/
Site of DARE database of diagnostic, and other, studies.

http://clinicalevidence.bmj.com/ceweb/index.jsp
Site of BMJ Clinical Evidence, an "authoritative medical resource for informing treatment decisions and improving patient care."

http://statpages.org/
Web pages, which are constantly updated, that perform statistical calculations; provides over 600 links, 380 "calculating pages," and a discussion on a range of power calculations.

Sources of Evidence

Evidence-Based Medicine journal
http://ebm.bmj.com/

National Library of Medicine, Health Services/Technology Assessment Text (HSTAT)
http://www.ncbi.nlm.nih.gov/books/bv.fcgi?rid=hstat

NHS Centre for Evidence-Based Medicine
http://www.cebm.net/

NHS Centre for Reviews and Dissemination
http://www.york.ac.uk/inst/crd/

ScHARR database (Netting the Evidence)
http://www.shef.ac.uk/scharr/ir/netting/

Sources of Guidelines

There are a large number of guideline databases that may also contain information regarding the use of tests in specific clinical situations. A selection is listed below.

Agency for Healthcare Research and Quality (AHRQ) U.S.
http://www.ahrq.gov

AGREE (Appraisal of Guidelines, Research, and Evaluation for Europe)
http://www.agreecollaboration.org

American Association of Clinical Endocrinologists
http://www.aace.com/pub/guidelines/

American College of Chest Physicians
http://www.chestnet.org/education/hsp/guidelinesProducts.php

American College of Physicians
http://www.acponline.org/clinical_information/guidelines/

CDC Guide to Community Preventive Services
http://www.thecommunityguide.org

Critical Efficacy Assessment Project (CEAP)
http://www.acponline.org/clinical_information/guidelines/process/ceap/

European Society of Cardiology
http://www.escardio.org/guidelines-surveys/esc-guidelines/Pages/GuidelinesList.aspx

German Agency for Quality in Medicine
http://www.aezq.de

Guideline Clearing House
http://guideline.gov

Guideline International Network (G-I-N)
http://www.g-i-n.net

Health Technology Organizations around the World
http://www.shef.ac.uk/scharr/ir/htaorg.html

The International Network of Agencies for Health Technology Assessment
http://www.inahta.org/INAHTA

National Academy of Clinical Biochemistry
Laboratory Medicine Practice Guidelines
http://www.aacc.org/members/nacb/LMPG/Pages/default.aspx

National Institute for Health Research, Health Technology Assessment Programme
http://www.ncchta.org/

National Kidney Foundation: Kidney Disease Outcomes Quality Initiative
http://www.kidney.org/Professionals/Kdoqi/guidelines

New Zealand Guidelines Group
http://www.nzgg.org.nz

NHS National Institute for Health and Clinical Excellence
http://www.nice.org.uk/guidance/index.jsp

ScHARR database (Netting the Evidence)
http://www.shef.ac.uk/scharr/ir/netting/

Scottish Intercollegiate Guidelines Network
http://www.sign.ac.uk/

Additional Reading

Armstrong EC. The well-built clinical question: a key to finding the best evidence efficiently. WMJ 1999;98:25–8.

Dawes M, Davies P, Gray A, et al., eds. Evidence-Based Practice: A Primer for Health Care Professionals. Edinburgh: Churchill Livingstone, 1999:254pp.

Del Mar C, Doust J, Glasziou P. Clinical Thinking: Evidence, Communication and Decision-Making. Oxford: Blackwell Publishing BMJ Books, 2006:144pp.

Egger M, Davey Smith G, Altman DG, eds. Systematic Reviews in Health Care: Meta-Analysis in Context, 2nd ed. London: BMJ Books, 2001:487pp.

Galen RS, Gambino SR. Beyond Normality: The Predictive Value and Efficiency of Medical Diagnoses. New York, NY: John Wiley & Sons, 1975:237pp.

Glasziou P, Del Mar C, Salisbury J. Evidence-Based Practice Workbook, 2nd ed. Oxford: Blackwell Publishing BMJ Books, 2007:208pp.

Glasziou PP, Irwig L, Aronson JK. Evidence-Based Medical Monitoring: From Principles to Practice. Oxford: Blackwell Publishing BMJ Books, 2008:376pp.

Greenhalgh T. How to Read a Paper: The Basics of Evidence-Based Medicine, 3rd ed. London: BMJ Books, 2006:248pp.

Guyatt G, Rennie D, eds. User's Guide to the Medical Literature. A Manual for Evidence-Based Clinical Practice. Chicago: JAMA and Archive Journals, American Medical Association, 2002:706pp.

Heneghan C, Badenoch D. Evidence-based Medicine Toolkit, 2nd ed. Oxford: Blackwell Publishing BMJ Books, 2006:112pp.

Heneghan C, De Brun C, Pearce-Smith N. Searching Skills Toolkit. London: Wiley-Blackwell BMJ Books, 2009:120pp.

Knottnerus JA, Buntinx F, eds. The Evidence Base of Clinical Diagnosis, 2nd ed. London: Wiley-Blackwell BMJ Books, 2008:320pp.

McGovern DPB, Valori RM, Summerskill WSM, Levi M. Key Topics in Evidence-Based Medicine. Oxford: BIOS Scientific Publishers Ltd., 2001:160pp.

Mugford M, Vale L, Donaldson C. Evidence-based Health Economics. London: BMJ Books, 2002:168pp.

Muir Gray JA. Evidence-Based Healthcare: How to Make Health Policy and Management Decisions, 2nd ed. Edinburgh: Churchill Livingstone, 2001:444pp.

Nordenström J. Evidence-Based Medicine in Sherlock Holmes' Footsteps. London: Blackwell Publishing, 2007:104pp.

Perera R, Heneghen C, Badenoch D. Statistics Toolkit. Oxford: Blackwell Publishing BMJ Books, 2008:120pp.

Price CP, Bossuyt PMM, Bruns DE. Introduction to laboratory medicine and evidence-based laboratory medicine. In: Burtis CA, Ashwood ER, Bruns DE, eds. Tietz Textbook of Clinical Chemistry and Molecular Diagnostics, 4th ed. Philadelphia: Elsevier Saunders, 2006:323–51.

Price CP, Christenson RH, eds. Evidence-Based Laboratory Medicine: Principles, Practice, and Outcomes, 2nd ed. Washington, DC: AACC Press, 2007:545pp.

Puglisi F, Federico E, Pertoldi B, Guerra S. Clinicians, diagnosis and clinical decision making: the importance of an evidence based approach. Part 1. Introduction to evidence based medicine and how to search for it. Adv Clin Path 2000;4:3–10.

Sackett DL, Haynes RB, Guyatt GH, Tugwell P. Clinical Epidemiology: A Basic Science for Clinical Medicine, 2nd ed. Toronto: Little, Brown, 1991:442pp.

Straus SE, Richardson WS, Glasziou P, Haynes RB. Evidence-Based Medicine: How to Practice and Teach EBM, 3rd ed. Edinburgh: Churchill Livingstone, 2005:320pp.

References

1. Knottnerus J, ed. The Evidence Base of Clinical Diagnosis. London: BMJ Books, 2002:226.

2. Collinson PO. The role of audit in laboratory medicine. In: Price CP, Christenson RH, eds. Evidence-Based Laboratory Medicine: Principles, Practice, and Outcomes, 2nd ed. Washington DC: AACC Press, 2007:347–73.

3. Strauss SE, Richardson WS, Glasziou P, Haynes RB. Evidence-Based Medicine. How to Teach and Practice EBM, 3rd ed. Edinburgh: Elsevier Churchill Livingstone, 2005:279–88.

4. Bandolier. Glossary index. Accessed November 5, 2008, at http://www.medicine.ox.ac.uk/bandolier/glossary.html.

5. Craig J, Bradbury I, Cummins E, Downie S, Foster L, Stout A. Health Technology Assessment Report 6. The use of B-type natriuretic peptides (BNP and NT-proBNP) in the investigation of patients with suspected heart failure. Glasgow, Scotland: NHS Quality Improvement, 2005. Accessed March 28, 2008, at http://www.nhshealthquality.org.

6. Boyd JC. Statistical analysis and presentation of data. In: Price CP, Christenson RH, eds. Evidence-Based Laboratory Medicine: Principles, Practice, and Outcomes, 2nd ed. Washington DC: AACC Press, 2007:113–40.

7. Moses LE, Shapiro D, Littenberg B. Combining independent studies of a diagnostic test into a summary ROC curve: data analytic approaches and some additional considerations. Statist Med 1993;12:1293–316.

8. Vamvakas EC. Meta-analysis of studies of the diagnostic accuracy of laboratory tests: a review of the concepts and methods. Arch Pathol Lab Med 1998;122:675–86.

9. Bossuyt PM, Reitsma JB, Bruns DE, et al. Towards complete and accurate reporting of studies of diagnostic accuracy: the STARD initiative. Clin Chem 2003;49:1–6.

10. Bossuyt PM, Reitsma JB, Bruns DE, et al. The STARD statement for reporting studies of diagnostic accuracy: explanation and elaboration. Clin Chem 2003;49:7–18.

11. Wikipedia. Validity. Accessed November 11, 2008, at http://en.wikipedia.org/wiki/Validity.

12. Jaeschke R, Guyatt GH, Sackett DL for the Evidence-Based Medicine Working Group. Users' guides to the medical literature. VI. How to use an article about a diagnostic test. B: What are the results and will they help me in caring for my patients? JAMA 1994;271:703–7.

13. Fagan TJ. Nomogram for Bayes theorem. N Engl J Med 1975;293:257.

14. Khunti K, Stone MA, Burden AC, et al. Randomized controlled trial of near patient testing for glycated haemoglobin in people with type 2 diabetes mellitus. Br J Gen Pract 2006;56:511–7.

Notes

Appendices

- Appendix A. Appropriate Study Design
- Appendix B. Classifying Levels of Evidence According to Type of Research Question
- Appendix C. CASP Critical Appraisal Checklist for Diagnostic Tests
- Appendix D. CASP Critical Appraisal Checklist for Prognostic Studies
- Appendix E. CASP Critical Appraisal Checklist for Outcome Studies
- Appendix F. Example of a Worked Critical Appraisal of Impact on Outcomes
- Appendix G. Generic Checklist for Applying Evidence (Step A4)
- Appendix H. Test Yourself

Appendix A

Appropriate Study Design

Best evidence develops by allowing the type of question (diagnostic, prognostic, etc.) to drive study design. For this reason, broadly classify the sort of question you are asking while you are formulating the question.

For example, in clinical medicine many important questions ask about interventions, therapies, or management strategies that are effective in treating a particular disease state. Also, the effectiveness of population screening for a given condition might be the topic of a clinical question that involves the impact of proposed screening programs.

In laboratory medicine, the clinical questions may be quite different. Many questions have to do with new technology and its ability to improve upon or replace existing technology by providing faster results, the same service at a lower cost, or a simpler, therefore more widely available, application. Further, many laboratory medicine questions involve diagnostic accuracy, including diagnostic sensitivity and specificity, for use in patients suspected of having a disease or condition. Other laboratory medicine questions address how a certain laboratory procedure predicts future outcomes, i.e., patient prognosis.

It is important to keep in mind that using tests to guide patient management or intervention in the diagnostic or monitoring process and improve outcomes (compared to no testing) is a most important utilization of laboratory medicine procedures. Clear examples of this use abound: for instance, utilization of rapid bedside glucose measurements in a comatose diabetic patient for deciding whether administering insulin (hyperglycemia) or glucose (hypoglycemia) is the appropriate treatment.

Pause and Reflect

Use the space below to give another example of how a laboratory test can guide patient management with a laboratory test.

....

....

....

Note that the type of study design is only one variable for determining the best evidence for answering clinical questions. This is because laboratory medicine fundamentally involves providing information to clinicians so that appropriate management decisions can be made for the individual patient. This is termed clinical effectiveness: i.e., "the right test, on the right patient, at the right time."

Effectiveness in Laboratory Medicine

The Right Test

For the Right Person

At the Right Time

Key Concept

Because the type of question (diagnostic, prognostic, etc.) drives study design, it is important to broadly classify the type of question you are asking while you are asking it. At the same time, remember the concept of clinical effectiveness: "the right test, for the right person, at the right time."

Matching Types of Study Design with Types of Questions

Cross-sectional vs. longitudinal design. Consider the case of a practitioner using a laboratory procedure for acute diagnosis of a condition such as hyperglycemia at a given moment in time. The practitioner uses an index test (glucose) which is performed and yields results nearly simultaneously with the outcome (the hyperglycemia diagnosis). This is an example of a *cross-sectional study*. It gives a snapshot that shows the outcome simultaneously with the test of interest. Other examples of cross-sectional studies include determining pregnancy with a POC hCG test, or the diagnosis of *Streptococcus* bacterial infection with a rapid Strep test in a practitioner's office.

The timing of test performance and the method of communicating the results for the "right test, collected at the right time" can have an important impact on patient management and outcome. Accounting in the study design for how and when the laboratory data are communicated to the responsible clinician can be a very important aspect of study design. There is always the question as to whether the clinician receives the result, makes the right decision, and takes the right action!

Longitudinal studies are when the index test is measured at one time and the outcome is measured or assessed at a later time. An example of a longitudinal study is the use of total cholesterol and HDL measurements, along with other Framingham risk variables (smoking status, age, gender, and blood pressure), to predict risk of coronary artery disease or death over the next ten years.

It is possible to use the same patient population in both cross-sectional and longitudinal studies. For example, cardiac troponin can be measured on the day of acute presentation and used for the purpose of diagnosing myocardial infarction (cross-sectional). The magnitude of increase in cardiac troponin can also be used to predict and stratify risk of death or re-infarction over the following year (longitudinal). The fact that cardiac troponin is positive can also be used to help guide use of therapies known to improve outcomes of acute coronary syndrome patients *(1)*. Thus, the cardiac troponin testing can be used for diagnosis, prognosis, and management.

Pause and Reflect

In the space below, list examples of cross-sectional and longitudinal studies in laboratory medicine specifying the index test and outcomes.

Cross-Sectional: ....

....

....

Longitudinal: ....

....

....

Randomized controlled trial design. In a randomized controlled trial (RCT) design, subjects are enrolled according to a set of criteria or characteristics so that all subjects are matched as closely as possible; this helps allow for experimental control of study conditions. The enrolled subjects are then randomized: i.e., they are assigned by chance to receive either the experimental treatment, intervention, or testing strategy under study, or the control treatment, intervention, or testing strategy.

Randomized Design

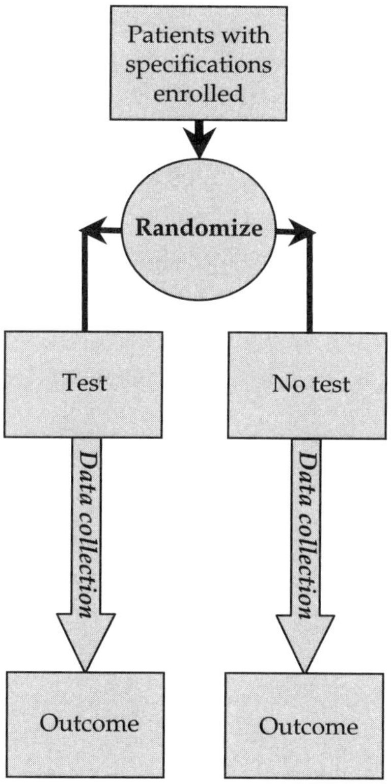

RCTs are longitudinal, prospective studies in which subjects are followed for the occurrence of outcomes. RCTs are often referred to as experimental studies because the randomization scheme determines which subjects receive the intervention, therapy, or test, and which subjects do not.

In laboratory medicine, a randomized design for availability of a new test to clinicians vs. a control arm where the test information is not available can help investigators assess the true impact of the test on outcomes. Alternatively, RCTs can compare existing tests having differing analytical sensitivities or specificities, or even availability of a point-of-care test for an analyte vs. measurement in the central laboratory. Again, outcomes must be followed to determine whether availability of the new test (or alternative test) has a significant effect. The outcomes can be health condition, differences in length of hospital stay, economic, etc.

RCTs are frequently considered a preferred study design because they minimize bias. However the enrollment criteria of subjects in a RCT must be carefully considered to assure they are not too restrictive and that the population studied matches your specific question. In other words, one must be cognizant of patient spectrum bias (see Part 3, Glossary).

Key Concepts

- RCT study design minimizes bias as long as the population studied matches the population referenced in the study question and that enrollment criteria are not overly restrictive.
- Outcomes from RCTs should be a result of incorporating information from the test. This assures that a clinical decision was made based on the result obtained, and one can evaluate the impact that the test had on the outcome(s).

Cohort study design. Cohort is a term derived from the Latin *Cohors*, which referred to a company of soldiers that were all of the same type, e.g., cavalry or infantry. A cohort of individuals shares one or more common characteristics such as occupation, weight, nation of origin, age, etc. (An inception cohort is a specific type of cohort in which the members have some commonality that caused them to be grouped together. An example would be the cohort of individuals who lived within 30 miles and were all exposed to radiation during the Chernobyl disaster.)

In healthcare, a cohort can be a group of patients, all of whom share the same age range and have similar signs and symptoms and care venue, e.g., primary care, urgent care, etc. Testing may be performed in some members of the cohort and not in others; thus decisions made using the added available information may lead to different outcomes in the tested cohort members. In contrast to an RCT, other than criteria at inception, cohort studies do not include a "control" of whether an intervention or test is administered to some but not to other members. For this reason cohort studies are considered "observational."

Cohort studies are often longitudinal, but depending on the question(s) under investigation, they can also be cross-sectional, or both. It is important to assure that the cohort in clinical studies matches the population relevant to your question. Audits (discussed in Step A5) and registries fall in the category of observational studies.

Diagnostic Accuracy Study Design. Questions that involve diagnostic sensitivity, specificity, positive predictive value, negative predictive value, and overall diagnostic accuracy are common in laboratory medicine. Diagnostic accuracy studies are cross-sectional and involve specifying a reference method or "gold standard," which is compared to the index test that is being evaluated. Subjects are enrolled in accordance with a cohort study design. The index test results are compared in the cohort to the reference method, usually using a 2 × 2 table (see figure below). Information from the 2 × 2 table allows calculation of diagnostic sensitivity, specificity, positive predictive value, negative predictive value, as well as overall diagnostic accuracy.

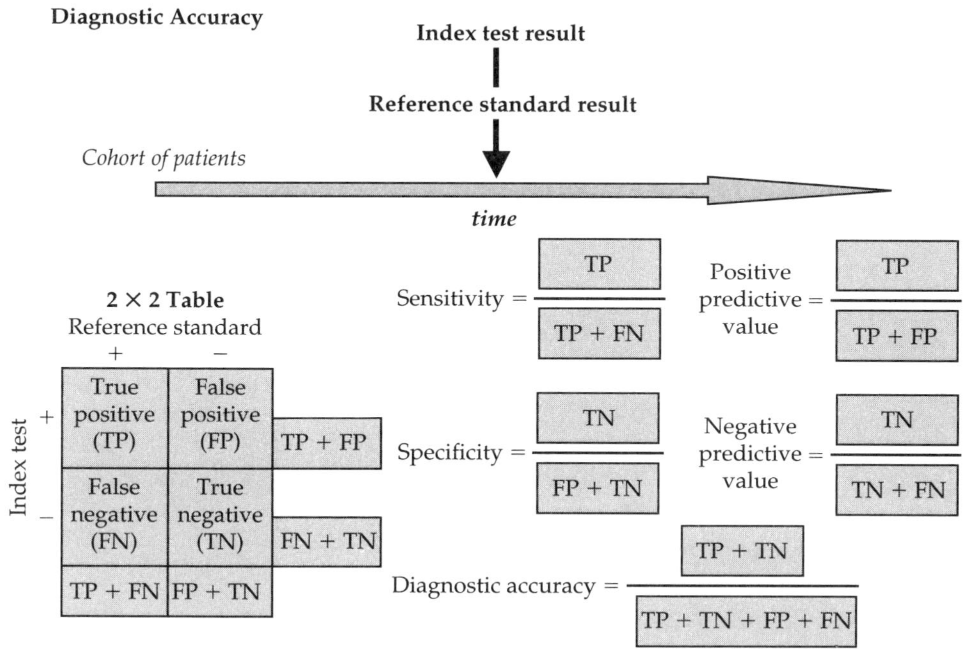

The characteristics of the cohort on which the new test is performed can have a profound impact on performance. Thus, to minimize patient spectrum bias, the study cohort must be matched as closely as possible with the population in your question in regard to severity of disease, prevalence of the target condition, timing of diagnosis (particularly for acute disease), and as many other factors as possible.

Application exercise: *A cohort of 1000 patients is being seen in a specialty rheumatoid arthritis (RA) clinic where the prevalence of RA is 50%. A new test for RA has a false positive rate of 3% and a false negative rate of 6%. Determine the diagnostic sensitivity, specificity, positive predictive value, negative predictive value, and diagnostic accuracy for the new test.*

Solution: *For the 1000-patient cohort in the rheumatoid arthritis clinic setting, 50% prevalence means that 500 patients have the RA diagnosis and 500 subjects are non-RA. Of the 500 RA patients, 470 have a true positive (TP) result for the test; 30 have a false negative (FN) result. For the non-RA subjects, 485 have a true negative (TN) result and 15 have a false positive (FP) result. The 2 × 2 table is as follows:*

New RA Test Result

Disease Diagnosis	*RA*	*Non-RA*	*Total*
Test positive	*TP 470*	*FP 15*	*TP + FP 485*
Test negative	*FN 30*	*TN 485*	*FN + TN 515*
	TP + FN 500	*FP + TN 500*	*Total 1000*

$$Sensitivity = \frac{470}{470 + 30} = 0.94; \ Specificity = \frac{485}{485 + 15} = 0.97$$

$$Positive\ predictive\ value = \frac{470}{470 + 15} = 0.959;$$

$$Negative\ predictive\ value = \frac{485}{485 + 30} = 0.942$$

$$Diagnostic\ accuracy = \frac{470 + 485}{1000} = 0.959$$

Pause and Reflect

Given the false positive and false negative rates above, how does diagnostic performance of the new RA test change if the test is performed in general practice office where the prevalence of RA is 10%, rather than 50%?

New RA Test Result

Disease Diagnosis	*RA*	*Non-RA*	*Total*
Test positive	*TP*	*FP*	*TP + FP*
Test negative	*FN*	*TN*	*FN + TN*
	TP + FN	*FP + TN*	*Total*

Sensitivity = ——— = ___________; *Specificity* = ——— = ___________

Positive predictive value = ——— = ___________

Negative predictive value = ——— = ___________

Diagnostic accuracy = ——— = ___________

What diagnostic parameters changed substantially? ....

....

....

Now check your work—solution available on page 237.

Prognostic study design. Questions involving a laboratory procedure's ability to predict (or prognosticate) outcomes are common in laboratory medicine. These questions involve a longitudinal cohort study design and are frequently termed "prognostic studies."

In prognostic studies a test is performed at a specified time and then the patient is followed for a specified interval to determine the outcome(s). Frequently Kaplan-Meier plots are used to indicate when outcomes occur, and odds ratios may be used to analyze test performance. Kaplan-Meier curves allow readers to easily compare and contrast different levels of different tests such as BNP and NT-proBNP and their impact on outcomes such as survival *(2)*. (Further information can be found in the critical appraisal section [see Part 2, Step A3]).

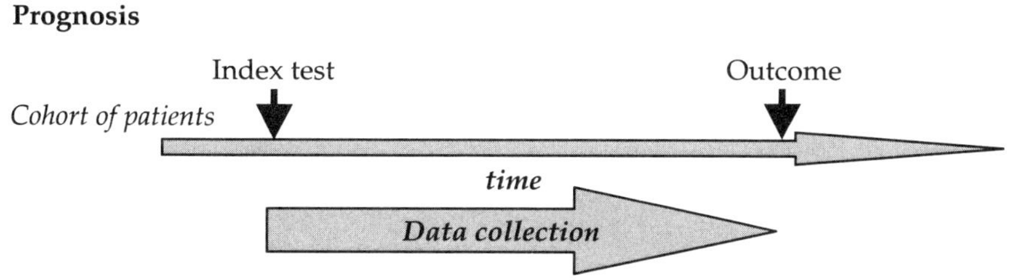

Case-control design. Case-control studies compare individuals who have an outcome such as development of a condition or disease (cases) to those who are part of the same initial cohort but who do not develop the outcome (controls). The controls are key to the study design; they should be from the initial cohort and must be matched as closely as possible to the cases in age, gender, life habits, comorbidities, etc. Case-control studies generally involve "looking back" longitudinally at an exposure or other variable that was different between the cases and matched controls to see if they might represent a risk factor or causative factor, or if there is an association of the variable with the outcome of interest.

Case control studies can be used in laboratory medicine to investigate a new biomarker that may indicate risk, i.e., for prognosis. Frequently, clinical trials have the foresight to place an enrollment specimen in a sample bank. This is useful if, for example, a new biomarker that might be useful for predicting the outcome of interest is discovered during the time of the study. With the passage of time, if some members of the cohort showed the outcome of interest (cases), while others from the inception cohort did not (controls), the new biomarker could be measured in enrollment samples of selected cases and matched controls. Analysis of differences in the biomarker between the cases and controls could be performed to see if the biomarker is predictive of the outcome of interest.

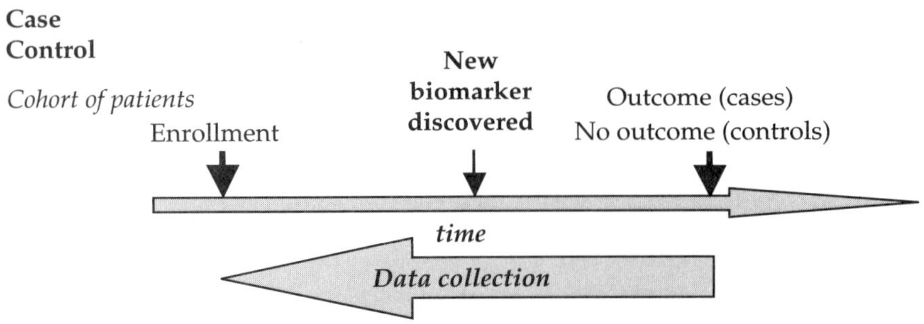

Before-and-after design (also known as before-after design) *(3)*. This is a descriptive term for a type of observational study that compares outcomes before a test is implemented and then after the test is implemented. Different populations of patients are frequently used for the before and after phases, although it is possible (but complicated) to use the same population in both the before and after phases. An example of such a study would be one that addresses the following question: *"Does availability of B-type natriuretic peptide (BNP) testing lead to earlier hospital discharge of congestive heart failure (CHF) patients admitted from the emergency department?"*

To address this question an investigator could monitor the length of hospital stay for a cohort of suspected CHF patients admitted from the emergency department before implementing BNP testing. Then, after a time during which an appropriate number of patients had been entered into the study, BNP testing would be implemented and the length of hospital stay documented for a similar cohort of suspected CHF patients. Then the length of stay for the "before" BNP cohort would be compared to the "after" BNP cohort.

Although this can be considered a valid study design, there are numerous potential problems that can be caused by changes over time in patient mix, changes in healthcare delivery, etc. Differences due to these changes, termed "secular trends," may be incorrectly attributed to the test intervention. To strengthen the before-and-after design, it may be possible to alternate access to the test, by turning "on" and then "off" availability for periods of time.

References

1. Morrow DA, Cannon CP, Jesse RL, et al. National Academy of Clinical Biochemistry Laboratory Medicine Practice Guidelines: Clinical characteristics and utilization of biochemical markers in acute coronary syndromes. Circulation 2007;115:e356–75.

2. deFilippi CR, Seliger SL, Maynard S, Christenson RH. Impact of renal disease on natriuretic peptide testing for diagnosing decompensated heart failure and predicting mortality. Clin Chem 2007;53:1511–9.

3. Guyatt G, Rennie D, Meade MO, Cook DJ. Users guide to the medical literature, 2nd ed. New York: McGraw-Hill Professional Publishing 2008:836pp.

Pause and Reflect Solution

Problem: *A new test for RA has a false positive rate of 3% and a false negative rate of 6%. Given the false positive and false negative rates above, how does diagnostic performance of the new RA test change if the test is performed in general practice office where the prevalence of RA is 10%, rather than 50%?*

Solution: *As in the worked example, having a 1000-patient cohort in the rheumatoid arthritis clinic setting is convenient. A prevalence of 10% means that 100 patients have the RA diagnosis, and 900 subjects are non-RA in this population. As before, the false negative rate is 6%, so 0.06 of the 100 patients = 6 false negatives; the remaining 94 are TPs. For the non-RA subjects, 0.97 of the 900 patients means that 873 have a TN result and 27 have a FP result. The new 10% prevalence 2 × 2 table is as follows:*

New RA Test Result

Disease Diagnosis	*RA*	*Non-RA*	*Total*
Test positive	*TP 94*	*FP 27*	*TP + FP 121*
Test negative	*FN 6*	*TN 873*	*FN + TN 879*
	TP + FN 100	*FP + TN 900*	*Total 1000*

From the 2 × 2 Table:

$$\textit{Sensitivity} = \frac{94}{94 + 6} = 94\%; \quad \textit{Specificity} = \frac{873}{873 + 27} = 97\%$$

$$\textit{Positive predictive value} = \frac{94}{94 + 27} = 0.777;$$

$$\textit{Negative predictive value} = \frac{873}{873 + 6} = 0.993$$

$$\textit{Diagnostic accuracy} = \frac{94 + 873}{1000} = 0.967$$

What diagnostic parameters changed substantially?

Positive predictive value dropped by almost 20%! Negative predictive value increased by about 5%. Diagnostic accuracy changed by less than 1%, and sensitivity and specificity (of course) did not change at all.

Thus the proportion of true positive results a test yields is very dependent on the prevalence of the disease in the population tested. The negative predictive value increases, but modestly by comparison.

Appendix B

Classifying Levels of Evidence According to Type of Research Question

For evidence to minimize bias and be of high quality, the design of the trial must match the type of question (see table). It is noteworthy that the most valuable laboratory procedures involve guidance of interventions or therapies known to improve patient outcome; these applications frequently involve designing randomized controlled trials to establish the value (economic and/or health outcome) of having the test information available for clinical decision making.

Evidence level		Diagnositic[1] question	Prognostic[2] question	Outcome question
Least biased	I	Systematic review of level II studies	Systematic review of level II studies	Systematic review of level II studies
↓	II	Cross-sectional study among consecutive presenting patients	Inception cohort study	Randomized controlled trial
↓	III	One of the following: – cross-sectional study among nonconsecutive patients – diagnostic case-control study, before-and-after study	One of the following: – untreated control patients in a randomized controlled trial – retrospectively assembled cohort study	One of the following: – cohort study design – case-control study
Most biased	IV	Case series	Case series, or a cohort study of patients at different stages of disease	Case series

[1] These levels of evidence apply only to studies of diagnostic accuracy. To assess the *effectiveness* of a diagnostic test, there also needs to be a consideration of the impact of the test on patient management and health outcomes.

[2] In rare instances, "all-or-none" evidence may be available for these types of questions and, depending on the circumstances, it may provide confirmation of effectiveness or causation.

Source: Modified from the Centre for Evidence-Based Medicine (Oxford) website (http://www.cebm.net/levels_of_evidence.asp) and the National Health and Medical Research Council (Australia) (http://www.nhmrc.gov.au).

Appendix C

CASP Critical Appraisal Checklist for Diagnostic Tests

Critical appraisal checklist from CASP (Critical Appraisal Skills Programme) for diagnostic tests. http://www.phru.nhs.uk/Pages/PHD/resources.htm (Accessed December 19, 2008). Explanatory notes are in brackets [...].

Adapted with permission from Public Health Resource Unit, NHS. Critical Appraisal Skills Programme (CASP). Making sense of evidence. 12 questions to help you make sense of a diagnostic test study. Oxford: Public Health Resource Unit, 2006:1–4. © Public Health Resource Unit, England (2006). All rights reserved.
and Jaeschke R, Guyatt G, Sackett DL. Users' guides to the medical literature. III. How to use an article about a diagnostic test. A. Are the results of the study valid? Evidence-Based Medicine Working Group. JAMA 1994;271:389–91.

A. Are the results of the study valid?			
Screening questions			
1. Was there a clear question for the study to address? *HINT: A question should include information about* • *the population.* • *the test.* • *the setting.* • *the outcomes.*	**Yes** ❑	**Can't tell** ❑ [Clear question formulation?]	**No** ❑
2. Was there a comparison with an appropriate reference standard? *HINT: Is this reference test(s) the best available indicator in the circumstances?*	**Yes** ❑	**Can't tell** ❑ [Gold standard appropriate?]	**No** ❑
Is it worth continuing?			
3. Did all patients get the diagnostic test and the reference standard? *HINT:* • *Were both received regardless of the results of the test of interest?* • *Check the 2 × 2 table (verification bias).*	**Yes** ❑	**Can't tell** ❑ [Verification bias present?]	**No** ❑

Continued

4. Could the results of the test of interest have been influenced by the results of the reference standard?

HINT:
- *Was there blinding?*
- *Were the tests performed independently? (review bias)*

Yes	Can't tell	No
❑	❑	❑
	[Review bias present?]	

5. Is the disease status of the tested population clearly described?

HINT:
- *presenting symptoms*
- *disease stage or severity*
- *co-morbidity*
- *differential diagnoses (spectrum bias)*

Yes	Can't tell	No
❑	❑	❑
	[Spectrum bias present?]	

6. Were the methods for performing the test described in sufficient detail?

HINT:
- *Was a protocol followed?*

Yes	Can't tell	No
❑	❑	❑
	[Design & conduct]	

Is it worth continuing?

B. If so, what are the results?

7. What are the results?

HINT: Consider
- *Are the sensitivity and specificity and/or likelihood ratios presented?*
- *Are the results presented in such a way that we can work them out?*

8. How sure are we about these results?

HINT: Consider
- *Could they have occurred by chance?*
- *Are there confidence limits?*
- *What are they?*

C. Will the results help me and my patients/population?

(Consider whether you are primarily interested in the impact on a population or individual level)

9. Can the results be applied to your patients/population of interest?

HINT:
Do you think your patients are/population is so different from those in the study that the results cannot be applied (such as age, sex, ethnicity, and spectrum bias)?

Yes	Can't tell	No
❑	❑	❑
	[Are the results relevant?]	

10. Can the test be applied to your patients/population of interest? *HINTS: Think of* • *resources and opportunity costs* • *level and availability of expertise required to interpret the tests* • *current practice and availability of service*	**Yes** ❑	**Can't tell** ❑ [Transferability?]	**No** ❑
11. Were all outcomes important to the individual or population considered? *HINT:* • *Will the knowledge of the test results improve patient wellbeing?* • *Will this knowledge of the test results lead to a change in patient management?*	**Yes** ❑	**Can't tell** ❑ [Outcome documented?]	**No** ❑
12. What would be the impact of using this test on your patients/population? [Impact of study on clinical care?]			

Appendix D

CASP Critical Appraisal Checklist for Prognostic Studies

Critical appraisal checklist from CASP (Critical Appraisal Skills Programme) for a cohort study appropriate for evaluating prognostic studies. http://www.phru.nhs.uk/Pages/PHD/resources.htm (Accessed December 19, 2008).

A. Are the results of the study valid?			
Screening questions			
1. Did the study address a clearly focused issue? *HINT: A question can be focused in terms of* • *the population studied* • *the risk factors studied* • *the outcomes considered* • *whether it is clear the study tried to detect a beneficial or harmful effect*	**Yes** ❑	**Can't tell** ❑	**No** ❑
2. Did the authors use an appropriate method to answer their question? *HINT: Consider* • *Is a cohort study a good way of answering the question under the circumstances?* • *Did it address the study question?*	**Yes** ❑	**Can't tell** ❑	**No** ❑
Is it worth continuing?			
3. Was the cohort recruited in an acceptable way? *HINT: We are looking for selection bias that might compromise the generalizability of the findings.* • *Was the cohort representative of a defined population?* • *Was there something special about the cohort?* • *Was everybody included who should have been included?*	**Yes** ❑	**Can't tell** ❑	**No** ❑

4. Was the exposure accurately measured to minimize bias? *HINT: We are looking for measurement or classification bias.* • *Did they use subjective or objective measurements?* • *Do the measures truly reflect what you want them to (have they been validated)?* • *Were all the subjects classified into exposure groups using the same procedure?*	**Yes** ❑	**Can't tell** ❑	**No** ❑
5. Was the outcome accurately measured to minimize bias? *HINT: We are looking for measurement or classification bias.* • *Did they use subjective or objective measurements?* • *Do the measures truly reflect what you want them to (have they been validated)?* • *Has a reliable system been established to detect all the cases (for measuring disease occurrence)?* • *Were the measurement methods similar in the different groups?* • *Were the subjects and/or the outcome assessor blinded to exposure (does this matter)?*	**Yes** ❑	**Can't tell** ❑	**No** ❑
6A. Have the authors identified all important confounding factors? List the ones the authors missed that you think might be important. **B. Have they considered the confounding factors in the design and/or analysis?** *HINT:* • *Look for restriction in design and techniques, e.g., modeling and stratified, regression, or sensitivity analysis to correct, control, or adjust for confounding factors.*	**Yes** ❑ **Yes** ❑ List:	**Can't tell** ❑ **Can't tell** ❑	**No** ❑ **No** ❑

Continued

7A. Was the follow-up of subjects complete enough?	**Yes** ❑	**Can't tell** ❑	**No** ❑
B. Was the follow-up of subjects long enough? *HINT:* • *The good or bad effects should have had long enough to reveal themselves.* • *The persons who are lost to follow-up may have different outcomes than those available for assessment.* • *In an open or dynamic cohort, was there anything special about the outcome of the people leaving or the exposure of the people entering the cohort?*	**Yes** ❑	**Can't tell** ❑	**No** ❑
B. What are the results?			
8. What are the results of this study? *HINT:* • *What are the bottom-line results?* • *Have they reported the rate or the proportion between the exposed/unexposed, the ratio/the rate difference?* • *How strong is the association between exposure and outcome (RR)?* • *What is the absolute risk reduction (ARR)?*	**9. How precise are the results?** **How precise is the estimate of the risk?** *HINT:* • *Size of the confidence intervals*		
10. Do you believe the results? *HINT:* • *A big effect is hard to ignore.* • *Can it be due to bias, chance, or confounding?* • *Are the design and methods of this study sufficiently flawed to make the results unreliable?* • *Consider Bradford Hills criteria (e.g., time sequence, dose-response gradient, biological plausibility, consistency).*	**Yes** ❑	**Can't tell** ❑	**No** ❑

C. Will the results help me locally?			
11. Can the results be applied to the local population? *HINTS: Consider whether* • *the subjects covered in the study could be sufficiently different from your population to cause concern.* • *your local setting is likely to differ much from that of the study.* • *Can you quantify the local benefits and harms?*	**Yes** ❑	**Can't tell** ❑	**No** ❑
12. Do the results of this study fit with other available evidence?	**Yes** ❑	**Can't tell** ❑	**No** ❑

Appendix E

CASP Critical Appraisal Checklist for Outcome Studies

Critical appraisal checklist from CASP (Critical Appraisal Skills Programme) for outcome studies. Explanatory notes are in brackets [...].

Adapted with permission from Public Health Resource Unit, NHS. Critical Appraisal Skills Programme (CASP). Making sense of evidence. 10 questions to help you make sense of randomised controlled trials. Oxford: Public Health Resource Unit, 2006:1–4. © Public Health Resource Unit, England (2006). All rights reserved. and Guyatt GH, Sackett DL, Cook DJ. Users' guides to the medical literature. II. How to use an article about therapy or prevention. A. Are the results of the study valid? Evidence-Based Medicine Working Group. JAMA 1993;270:2598–601. and Guyatt GH, Sackett DL, Cook DJ. Users' guides to the medical literature. II. How to use an article about therapy or prevention. B. What were the results and will they help me in caring for my patients? Evidence-Based Medicine Working Group. JAMA 1994;271:59–63.

A. Are the results of the study valid?	
Screening questions	
1. Was there a clear question for the study to address? *HINT: A question should include information about* • *the population* • *the test* • *the setting* • *the outcomes*	**Yes** ❑ **Can't tell** ❑ **No** ❑ [Clear question formulation?]
2. Was the intervention compared with a control group in a way that minimized bias, and yet ensured that the results were used to make clinical decisions leading to an outcome? *HINT: Was the new test part of an explicit decision-making process that was followed, and was this compared with the current decision-making process?*	**Yes** ❑ **Can't tell** ❑ **No** ❑ [Intervention compared with control?]
Is it worth continuing?	
3. Were participants clearly identified and appropriately allocated to intervention and control group? *HINT:* • *Was the process truly random?* • *Was the process described?* • *Are there any differences between the groups at entry?* • *If there were differences, might they have explained any outcomes (confounding)?*	**Yes** ❑ **Can't tell** ❑ **No** ❑ [Verification bias present?]

4. Were participants, staff, and study personnel "blind" to participant's study group? *HINT:* • *Was an effort made to achieve blinding?* • *Blinding may not be possible.* • *Was there any evidence of operator or observer bias?*	**Yes** ❑	**Can't tell** ❑ [Review bias present?]	**No** ❑
5. Were all of the participants who entered the trial accounted for at its conclusion? *HINT:* • *Did all participants meet the criteria for whom test was intended?* • *Did any participants find their way into the other group?* • *Were any participants lost to follow-up?*	**Yes** ❑	**Can't tell** ❑ [Spectrum bias present?]	**No** ❑
6. Were the methods for performing the tests described, enough participants recruited, participants followed-up, and data collected in the same way? *HINT:* • *Was a protocol followed for both intervention and control arms?* • *Were sufficiently robust outcome measures employed in the study?* • *Was there a power calculation?* • *Were all participants tested and monitored in the same way, at the same time intervals?*	**Yes** ❑	**Can't tell** ❑ [Design & conduct; performance bias present?]	**No** ❑
Is it worth continuing?			
B. If so, what are the results?			
7. How are the results presented and what is the main result? *HINT:* • *Were the correct statistical tools used?* • *Are the results presented in such a way that we can work them out?* • *How large is the size of the result and is it meaningful?*			

Continued

8. How precise are these results? *HINT:* • *Is the result precise enough to make a decision?* • *Are confidence limits reported?* • *Are p-values reported?*	

C. Will the results help me and my patients/population?
(Consider whether you are primarily interested in the impact on a population or individual level.)

9. Can the results be applied to your patients/population of interest? *HINT:* • *Do you think your patients are/population is so different from those in the study that the results cannot be applied (such as age, sex, ethnicity, and spectrum bias)?* • *Is your patient/population setting different from that of the trial, e.g., primary vs. secondary care?*	**Yes** ❑ **Can't tell** ❑ **No** ❑ [Are the results relevant?]
10. Can the test be applied to your patient or population of interest? *HINTS: Think of* • *resources and opportunity costs* • *level and availability of expertise required to interpret the tests* • *current practice, change of practice, and availability of service*	**Yes** ❑ **Can't tell** ❑ **No** ❑ [Transferability?]
11. Were all outcomes important to the individual or population considered? *HINT:* • *Will the knowledge of the test results improve patient well-being?* • *Will this knowledge of the test results lead to a change in patient management?* • *Will it be possible to make the required change in patient management?* • *Were any risks associated with adopting the approach taken in the trial explored and are they relevant to your situation?*	**Yes** ❑ **Can't tell** ❑ **No** ❑ [Outcome documented?]

12. What would be the impact of using this test on your patients/population?
[Impact of study on clinical care?]

Appendix F

The paper being considered, available free at http://care.diabetesjournals.org/cgi/reprint/22/11/1785, is the study by Cagliero et al. *(1)*.

Example of a Worked Critical Appraisal of Impact on Outcomes

Patient population: Patients with diabetes (types 1 and 2) being managed in a secondary outpatient clinic.

Intervention/Test: POCT for HbA1c with feedback delivered immediately.

Comparator/Control: Central laboratory delivery of HbA1c test results.

Outcome: Change in HbA1c levels (using a laboratory method).

The next step is to work through the outcomes checklist; this checklist is designed for critical appraisal of randomized controlled trials. It was written in such a way that one can evaluate the validity of a before-and-after study design as well.

> Note: This study was conducted in a secondary care diabetes clinic, so it is a good example of using the PICOS approach to question formulation, where "S" is for "setting." Note also the comments at point 12 on page 253, which relate to a similar study in a primary care setting. But was it similar?

Screening questions:

1. *Was there a clear question for the study to address?*

   In the introduction to the paper *(1)*, one stated aim was to *". . . [test] the hypothesis that HbA1c results available at the time of physician encounter could improve glucose control by changing physician and/or patient behavior."*

   Response: Yes

> The question should contain the population, the intervention (test), the control (test), the setting and the outcome.

2. *Was the intervention compared with a control group in a way that minimized bias, yet ensured that the results were used to make clinical decisions leading to an outcome?*

   The "Research Design and Methods" section of the paper stated *"Patients were randomly assigned to one of two groups: one group had HbA1c levels determined at the time of the office visit with the benchtop analyzer so that results of the HbA1c test were available to the individual*

> Was the study a randomized controlled trial (as this is the best approach to minimizing bias)? Note: It has been suggested that a before-and-after study design would be an alternative approach to testing the impact of diagnostic tests on health outcomes.

physicians at the beginning of the visit (immediate assay group), and the other had HbA1c levels measured by the diabetes laboratory as per usual clinical practice (control group)."

Response: Yes

Is it worth continuing?

Response: Yes; the response to both screening questions is yes.

3. *Were participants clearly identified and appropriately allocated to intervention and control groups?*

In the "Research Design and Methods" section, the patients were identified as type 1 diabetics and insulin-treated type 2 diabetics. All patients were randomly assigned to one of two groups as noted earlier. No further details of the randomization were given. However, when considering what factors might influence the outcomes, it was noted in the results section that the proportion of patients with type 1 diabetes was similar for both groups, as was the number of insulin doses and injections per day.

Response: Yes. The "Represent" and "Allocation" aspects of **RA**MMbo were appropriate.

Intention-to-treat analysis is intended to avoid misrepresentation in intervention research studies. Intention to treat is based on the subject's initial assignment, not on the intervention actually administered. For the purpose of intention-to-treat analysis, all subjects who are assigned to receive the intervention are considered to be part of the trial and their outcomes count, whether they drop out or not.

4. *Were participants, staff, and study personnel "blind" to participants' study group?*

The "Research Design and Methods" section stated *"The patients were treated by staff physicians and endocrinology fellows; the physicians were aware of the nature of the study (clinical evaluation of immediate HbA1c assay) but were masked to the specific outcomes collected (e.g., frequency of visits, changes in therapy, contacts with patients) . . ."* It is almost impossible to blind the physicians completely as they will be adopting a different form of practice (maybe unknowingly—and this is part of the study's objectives) depending on which group the patient is allocated to, and in this instance he/she will be aware of dealing with a current result for the HbA1c or an earlier result—although that result will no doubt have been communicated to the patient in some way.

Response: Blinding was part of the study design. The "blinded" aspect of RAMM**b**o was adequate.

Was there blinding? (Look for observer or operator bias.)

5. *Were all of the participants who entered the trial accounted for at its conclusion?*

From Table 1 and the "Results" section: Of the 201 patients recruited, 37 did not complete the study (14/100 in the immediate assay group and 23/101 in the control group). One patient died, seven were lost to follow-up, and 23 did not have a HbA1c result measured within the last six months of the study—necessary as HbA1c was one of the outcome measures.

Response: The "Maintenance" aspect of RA**M**Mbo was adequately covered.

Results of the intervention group can be misleading if subjects who have a lower response to the intervention or more serious disease drop out of the study at a higher rate, because then only the subjects assigned to the intervention group for whom the treatment worked will be analyzed. Thus ineffective interventions may appear to provide benefit if only the intervention subjects who finish the study are compared with controls.

This is why all the participants who entered the trial must be accounted for at its conclusion.

6. *Were the methods for performing the tests described, enough participants recruited, participants followed-up, and data collected in same way?*

The analytical methods in the study are well described for both the intervention and control arms, with performance of both described in an earlier pilot study to assess analytical performance. The primary outcome was a change in the HbA1c result measured using the laboratory method over the one-year study period. According to the paper: "The secondary outcomes included changes in insulin therapy, hypoglycemic episodes, and use of health care resources as determined by patient questionnaires and chart reviews." The only stated difference between the two arms of the study was that the physicians in the intervention arm had current HbA1c results available for immediate feedback of results. However, the possibility of operator bias must be kept in mind because the physicians knew they were participating in a trial to assess the effectiveness of having an immediate HbA1c result. There was no power calculation.

Response: The "Measurement" and "Objective" aspects of RAMM**b**o were appropriate.

(i) Was a protocol followed for both the intervention and control arms?

(ii) Were sufficiently robust outcome measures employed in the study?

(iii) Was there a power calculation?

(iv) Were all participants tested and monitored in the same way, at the same time intervals?

Is it worth continuing?

Response: Yes

7. *How are the results presented and what is the main result?*

In the study, the changes in the HbA1c results at 6 and 12 months after entry were presented graphically for the two groups against the baseline values (mean ± SEM) with the data also described in the text. HbA1c levels fell significantly in the immediate assay group (by 0.51 ± 1.44% at 6 months [p=0.001] and by 0.41 ± 1.65% at 12 months [p=0.013]), but not in the control group (by 0.11 ± 0.79% at 6 months [not significant] and 0.19 ± 1.16% at 12 months [not significant]).

Response: The results were reported in a clear and helpful way.

(i) Were the correct statistical tools used?

(ii) Are the results presented in such a way that we can work them out?

(iii) How large is the size of the result and is it meaningful?

8. *How precise are these results?*

Response: The number of patients included in the trial was 164. There was no power calculation performed. Although the study may have been underpowered for detecting a statistically significant difference at 6 months, the change in HbA1c levels at 6 months and one year in the immediate group were significant as judged against the baseline values.

(i) Is the result precise enough to make a decision?

(ii) Are there confidence limits reported?

(iii) Are p-values reported?

9. *Can the results be applied to your patients/the population of interest?*

Response: The results can be generalized to type 2 diabetics treated in a secondary care setting. You may wish to consider other studies to broaden the applicability of these findings to different populations—e.g., non-insulin dependent diabetics.

(i) Do you think your patients are/population is so different from those in the study that the results cannot be applied? (Hint: Consider age, sex, ethnicity, and spectrum bias)

(ii) Is your patient/population setting different from that of the trial, e.g., primary vs. secondary care?

10. *Can the test be applied to your patient or population of interest?*

Response: The analytical performance of the POCT is comparable with that of the laboratory. The three main considerations when introducing a POCT service are (i) the shifting of resources as it is generally the case that the costs of providing the POCT service will be greater than those of the laboratory; (ii) the training and quality assurance requirements to ensure that the quality of the analytical result can be maintained; and (iii) the change in clinical practice required in order for the POCT service to generate the results seen in this study—primarily a change in the style of the consultation with the patient in order to make the best use of the immediate HbA1c result. The study did not show any significant reduction in short-term costs of care, e.g., clinic visits, calls to

Consider resources and opportunity costs, training, QA requirements, and expertise needed for test interpretation, and availability of services.

patients, etc., although they did recognize that there was a long-term cost benefit from a 0.5% reduction in the HbA1c level. It is worth noting that this study outcome was achieved over a period of one year, and so further work would be needed to determine (i) if, and how, this benefit could be maintained over a number of years, and (ii) the health outcome benefit of maintaining this improvement over a number of years.

11. *Were all outcomes important to the individual or population considered?*

Response: There was a significant improvement in the HbA1c levels in the immediate assay group; HbA1c is a recognized surrogate outcome marker of morbidity and mortality in patients with diabetes. The use of POCT was associated with a change in management—that was part of the study hypothesis—namely, immediate feedback of the HbA1c result. The analytical performance of the POCT system is the same as the laboratory method and so it is unlikely that performance characteristics will have an impact on adverse outcomes, as long as the operators are trained properly and participate in quality management procedures. There was no increase in untoward incidents, e.g., hypoglycemic episodes or emergency hospital admissions, associated with use of the POCT service.

(i) Will knowledge of the test results improve patient well-being?

(ii) Will this knowledge of the test results lead to a change in patient management?

(iii) Will it be possible to make the required change in patient management?

(iv) Were any risks associated with adopting the approach taken in the trial explored and are they relevant to your situation?

12. *What would be the impact of using this test on your patients/population?*

Response: The patient population described in the study that was appraised matched closely with that of the originator of the question. However, it is important to appreciate that it may not be generalizable to all populations and settings, e.g., in non-insulin dependent diabetics and to primary care. A recent study covering these two scenarios, however, points to another vitally important point when appraising a study. Khunti et al. *(2)* performed a randomized controlled trial in primary care and found no difference in the HbA1c results. However, in the discussion of their results, the authors indicated that they did not change their practice—i.e., they did not use the POCT approach to engage in immediate feedback of the results for use in the interaction of the physician with the patient.

Note: This study was conducted in a primary care setting. In the discussion you will read that "In practice it proved difficult for surgeries to organize their management of patients … in such a way as to maximize the benefits of using the rapid test … Practices therefore often continued their follow-up in the usual way." It seems these authors did not change their practice to take advantage of rapid testing and immediate patient feedback. So, the studies were not similar.

References

1. Cagliero E, Levina E, Nathan D. Immediate feedback of HbA1c levels improves glycemic control in type 1 and insulin-treated type 2 diabetic patients. Diabetes Care 1999;22:1785–9.

2. Khunti K, Stone MA, Burden AC, et al. Randomized controlled trial of near patient testing for glycated haemoglobin in people with type 2 diabetes mellitus. Br J Gen Pract 2006;56:511–7.

Appendix G

Generic Checklist for Applying Evidence (Step A4)

P: Is the patient (or population) similar to that described in the study?

- *Does the patient (or population) with whom you are now concerned match those described in the study? Important factors to consider: age, sex, ethnicity, stage in the evolution of the condition, severity of condition.*
- *Are the patients (or population) featured in the study so different from those with whom you are concerned that the study results are not applicable to your population or patient?*
- *Is the setting of the study comparable to the setting in the question posed (e.g., primary or secondary care)?*
- *Are the reference ("normal") ranges quoted in the study comparable with those in the situation of concern?*
- *Are the action limits (if relevant) quoted in the study appropriate to the situation with which you're concerned?*

> Remember, we suggested you use "S" for "setting" when designing your PICO. The importance of "setting" is likely to be reflected in the use of diagnostic tests, more so than in other interventions, as it is likely to reflect different stages in the disease. An example would be when comparing the use of natriuretic peptide measurements in primary care with those in secondary care, and even between scenarios within the latter, e.g., patients presenting for hospital admission, to the emergency department, or to urgent care.

I: Is the new analytical test method well described and correctly validated?

- *Has the accuracy of the new test method been validated?*
- *Has the precision of the new test method been validated?*
- *Are the analytical performance characteristics of the new test method (e.g., accuracy, precision, and the diagnostic accuracy performance characteristics) comparable with the comparator method—and appropriate?*
- *Is there any evidence that the analytical performance of the new test method (i.e., accuracy and precision) has any impact on the health outcome (e.g., on the nature of the clinical decisions that will be made)?*
- *Do the problems addressed in the study match those posed by your question, or that of the inquirer?*

C: Is the comparator test method well described and correctly validated?

- *Has the accuracy of the comparator test method been validated?*
- *Has the precision of the comparator test method been validated?*
- *Are the diagnostic accuracy performance characteristics of the comparator method well described—either in the paper, or in referenced literature (e.g., is there a recognized "gold standard")?*
- *Is there any evidence that the analytical performance of the comparator test method (i.e., its accuracy and precision) has any impact on the health outcome (e.g., on the nature of the clinical decisions that will be made)?*

Change management: What changes will be needed to gain the benefit?

Remember, we suggested you add "C" for "change management" when developing your PICO—especially when considering outcome studies. These are some of the questions you should be asking yourself when reviewing evidence, designing outcome studies to generate evidence, and when applying evidence.

Is there a clear vision of the benefits that will accrue from using the test in the way described in the study (i.e., what is the value proposition)?

- *What changes may have to be made to the process of care? e.g., consider*
  - *Change in diagnostic tests?*
  - *Change in operational aspects of delivery of the test?*
  - *Change in treatment protocol?*
  - *Change in monitoring the patient?*
- *What are the staff training and accreditation issues for the health professionals involved?*
- *Are there any risks for the patient?*
- *Are there any operational implications for the patient?*
- *How will the change be explained to the patient?*
- *What is the patient's view on the proposed change to practice?*
- *Is there an increase in financial expenditure involved with using the new test, and a saving to be made elsewhere in the organization(s) providing the package of care, or for the patient(s)?*
- *Who are the key personnel responsible for the departments and clinical groups involved in the change to the process of care?*
- *Are the changes identified deliverable?*

- *Will it be possible to reallocate resources in order to make the necessary operational changes to the process of care and deliver the benefits?*
- *What is the expected time to deliver the change and is there an implementation plan?*

Here are some of the big challenges of implementing change, which will impact your success in applying EBLM.

O: Are the outcome measures realistic and robust?

- *Are the outcome measures specifically stated and relevant?*
- *Is the time between testing and outcome assessment appropriate?*
- *Are the outcome measures described valid for this type of study application?*
- *Are the outcome measures used in the study applicable to the question being asked in the situation you are dealing with at the moment?*
- *Are the outcome measures used in the study assessed in the same way that you are considering? For example, will the length-of-stay identified in the study be applicable to your situation, and can the benefits be realized?*

Remember, if a test is to be made available to patients, it is important to demonstrate better outcomes (clinical, operational, or economic) if the test is to be of value.

Appendix H

Test Yourself

Use the T-chart below to summarize the key details of what you have learned about applying EBLM.

T-Chart: EBLM and the A5 Cycle	
Main ideas	**Key details or examples**
EBLM	
A1: Ask	
A2: Acquire	
A3: Appraise	
A4: Apply	
A5: Assess/Audit	

Suggested Answers to the T-Chart

T-Chart: EBLM and the A5 Cycle	
Main ideas	**Key details or examples/applications**
EBLM	• Evidence-based laboratory medicine • Best evidence for clinical decision making, focused on "foreground" rather than "background" information • Applications include analytical performance of tests, interpretation of test results, new applications of a test, tests and their impact on health outcomes, the use of tests in process change, and audit in relation to financial and clinical governance.
A1: Ask	How to form a structured question using the PICO approach: P: population I: intervention C: comparator [C]: change management O: outcome [S]: setting [T]: time
A2: Acquire	How to perform a search: See details about structured questions, using PubMed and other databases, and techniques and tips on pages 91–115.
A3: Appraise	Structured approach to evaluating evidence. Focus on • the primary clinical question • the relevance of evidence to the problem • potential biases such as appropriateness of the patient population • quality of the study's conduct Systematic review = most reliable evidence Be wary of confounders and bias.
A4: Apply	See if the evidence matches your clinical situation by asking questions such as the ones in Appendix G.
A5: Assess/Audit	Crucial to quality management Note role of change management Barth's five points (see p. 188)

Index

A

A5 cycle, 20, 43, 119, 177, 180
access to tests, 4*f*, 10
  outcomes and, 12
accuracy. *See also* analytical methods; diagnostic accuracy
  study description of, 161
  of study results, 158
  validation of, 151
ACP Journal Club, 96*t*
action limits, 151, 155, 161, 167
age, as confounder, 122
Agency for Healthcare Research and Quality (AHRQ) web address, 216
AGREE checklist, 21, 126*t*, 193, 215
albumin:creatinine ratio, 29, 58, 67
American Association for Clinical Chemistry, 86, 214
amino-terminal proBNP tests, 129–133. *See also* B-type natriuretic peptide tests
analytical methods
  evaluation of, 158
  performance assessment, 33, 161–162
  question formulation, 74–77
  study applicability and, 157–158
  study description of, 161–162
Annals of Clinical Biochemistry web address, 213
application process
  answering clinician questions, 24–31
  clinical situations and, 149–150
  review of performance, 186
Association for Clinical Biochemistry (U.K.), 86
attrition bias, definition, 193
audit
  clinical, definition, 194
  definition, 193
  of performance, 182–186
  process of, 188
  of processes, 32
  of utilization, 30

B

B-type natriuretic peptide tests
  application to practice, 157–160
  diagnostic performance questions, 63
  diagnostic question, 129–133
  evaluation of evidence in, 35–36
  evidence acquisition, 97–99, 113–114
  prognostic question, 133–137
  question formulation, 54–55
  resource utilization and, 83
  treatment decision questions and, 71–72
background information
  clinical laboratory information, 18
  description of, 7
  laboratory tests as, 11, 18
  questions related to, 46–47
Bandolier web address, 213
Bayes' theorem, 193, 208
before-and-after study, 193, 236
best evidence. *See also* evidence
  clinical decision making and, 7
  definition, 6
  selection of, 121
  study design and, 10
bias
  attrition, 193
  chance *versus*, 6
  confirmation, 195
  definition, 193
  differential verification, 196
  disease-progression, 196
  error and, 6
  evidence and, 121
  inappropriate-reference test, 198
  inclusion, 198
  incorporation, 198
  indexing, 198
  language, 198
  minimization of, 127–128, 135
  observer, 200
  operator, 200
  partial verification, 200
  performance, 200
  publication, 201
  review, 131, 202
  selection, 134, 203
  spectrum, 121, 132, 203
  threat of, 123
  verification, 131
biological variation, impact of, 18
blinding, 140, 194
BMC Medical Research Methodology web address, 213
BMJ web address, 213
Boolean search operators, 95*f*
  choice of, 99, 99*f*
  PubMed options, 100*t*, 108
breast cancer, prognostic tests, 66–67
business cases, 13, 19, 27–28, 39–40, 71, 75, 161, 181

C

C-reactive protein (CRP), 46–47, 66
calculations, 206–212
case-control study
  critical appraisal of, 124
  definition, 194
  questions answered by, 92*t*, 235
CASP checklist, 126*t*, 127–130, 194, 214
  in a BNP scenario, 130
  definition, 194
  for diagnostic tests, 239–241
  for outcome studies, 246–248
  for prognostic tests, 242–245
  in technology systematic review, 143–145
CAT (Critically Appraised Topic), 194
CEBM checklist, 127*t*
Centre for Evidence-Based Medicine, 86, 215
Centre for Health Evidence (CHE) web address, 215
chance, bias *versus*, 6
change management
  benefits and, 152–153, 163–164
  of changes in practice, 159–160
  review of performance, 187
  steps in, 159–160
changes in practice
  Chlamydia testing questions, 82
  decision making and, 70
  evidence application and, 149
  impact of evidence-based medicine, 20
  management of, 159–160
  PICO principle and (PICCO), 51, 153
  setting changes and, 51
  stakeholders in, 160, 164
CHE checklist, 127*t*, 215
checklists. *See also* AGREE, CASP, CEBM, and QUADAS checklists
  application of evidence, 255–257
  for applying evidence, 151–156
  use of, 126*t*
Chlamydia screening scenarios
  analytical performance questions, 79–80
  application of evidence to, 160–164
  economic outcome questions, 83–84
  evaluation of test effectiveness, 39–40
  resource allocation and, 82
cholesterol level scenario, 55
clinical audit, definition, 194
Clinical Chemistry web address, 213, 214
clinical decision analysis, 194
Clinical Evidence journal, 18
Clinical Evidence web address, 216
clinical outcomes. *See also* outcomes
  definition, 13
  measures of, 13
  surrogate measures of, 14*t*
clinical practice guideline, 194
clinical questions
  in daily practice, 182–186
  test ordering and, 18
clinicians, information needs, 24–27
The Cochrane Library, 96*t*, 216
cohort study
  comparator test method, 152
  confounders, 122
  critical appraisal of, 124
  definition, 195
  questions answered by, 92*t*, 232
  recruitment issues, 134
  relevance of, 134
colon neoplasia, 58–59
comorbidity, definition, 195
comparator test methods, 162
comparisons, evidence and, 149
confidence interval (CI), 195
confidence limits
  consideration of, 136–137
  reporting of, 132, 141, 145
confirmation bias, definition, 195
confounder variable
  awareness of, 122–123
  consideration of, 135–136
  definition, 195
congestive heart failure
  BNP questions, 129–137, 157–160
  evidence acquisition, 113–114
continuous variable, 195
controls
  evidence application and, 149
  in the PICO acronym, 8, 49–87, 97, 122, 149–153
cost-benefit analysis, definition, 195
cost-effectiveness analysis, definition, 195
cost-minimization analysis, definition, 195
cost-utility analysis, definition, 196
coumadin therapy monitoring, 79
critical appraisal process
  CASP checklist for, 239–241
  checklists, 126*t*–127*t*, 239–241
  definition, 120
  diagnostic applications, 129–133

of evidence, 119–146
impact on outcomes, 138–142, 249–254
key factors, 121–125
for methodological quality, 127–128
prognostic applications, 133–137
review of performance, 185
of a technology systematic review, 143–145
tools for, 126–128
cross-sectional study
definition, 196
longitudinal study *vs.*, 230
cystatin C scenario
diagnostic performance questions, 64
evaluation of new tests, 34–35

D

D-dimer testing
evidence acquisition, 103–111
technology systematic review, 143–145
databases
choice of, 97
for locating evidence, 95*t*–96*t*
selection of, 144
decision making
best evidence and, 7
changes in practice and, 70
elements of, 6–7
laboratory investigations and, 4*f*
patient-centered, 12
patient management and, 133
patient values and, 6–7
study design choice, 92*t*
treatment questions and, 71–72
use of test results, 26
dependent variable, definition, 196
diabetes-related scenarios, 58, 59. *See also* glycemic control; HbA1c point-of-care testing scenarios
diagnosis-related questions, 58, 62–65, 75
diagnostic accuracy, 234. *See also* QUADAS checklist
calculation of, 234, 237
of comparative test methods, 162
questions, 232–234
study of, 196
study design choice, 92*t*
diagnostic odds ratio (DOR), 196, 208
diagnostic performance, 210–212
diagnostic tests
critical appraisal of, 124
key objectives, 150*f*
dichotomous variable, definition, 196
differential verification bias, definition, 196
dipstick tests, settings for, 62
disease progression bias, definition, 196
diseases
etiology of, 54–57
laboratory tests and, 10
doctor-patient relationships, 45–48
Down syndrome, 75

E

economic outcomes
analytical performance questions, 74
in business case development, 27–28
change in practice and, 159–160
definition, 14
measures of, 14
question formulation, 82–88
test acceptance and, 164
effectiveness
of tests, 16
types of, 230
EMBASE, description, 96*t*
emergency department waiting-time scenarios
application of PICO to, 12
generic questions, 12
needs assessment in, 38–39
operational questions, 78–79
point-of-care testing and, 82–83
error
bias and, 6
definition of, 6
type I, 210–211
type II, 210–211
etiology of disease, questions, 54–57
evidence. *See also* best evidence
acquisition of, 89–115
application of, 32, 149–173, 255–257
assimilation of, 17
bias and, 121
checklists, 151–156
critical appraisal of, 119–146
databases containing, 95*t*–96*t*
definition, 6
dissemination of, 19
evaluation strategies, 18, 32
finding of, 32
generation of, 19
hierarchy of, 11*f*, 13*f*

evidence. *See also* best evidence *(Continued)*
integration with experience, 6
internet sources of, 217
levels of, 238
outcomes assessment and, 19
secondary research sources, 94
evidence-based healthcare, definition, 196
evidence-based journals, 18
evidence-based laboratory medicine (EBLM)
A5 cycle for, 20, 43, 119, 177, 180
assimilation of, 180
audit process in, 188, 188*f*
cycle of, 188*f*
day-to-day practice of, 21–23
definition, 10, 197
glossary, 193–205
key challenges of, 3–5
lifelong learning and, 177–181
overview, 10–14
professional associations, 86
roots of, 4
skills needed, 21–23
evidence-based medicine (EBM)
definitions, 4, 197
evolution of, 17, 18
Evidence-Based Medicine (Strauss), 17
exclusion criteria, definition, 197
experience
clinical judgment and, 17
evidence integrated with, 6
external validity, 150, 197

F

Fagan nomogram, 49, 208–209
fasting blood sugar screening, 59
fixed-effect model, 197
foreground information
description of, 7
investigative studies, 18
need for, 18
questions related to, 46–47

G

gender, as confounder, 122, 123
gene profiling, prognostic performance, 66–67
glossary, 193–205
glycemic control scenarios. *See also* HbA1c point-of-care testing scenarios
analytical performance questions, 74
evaluation of method performance, 33–34
point-of-care testing and, 138–142
treatment decision questions, 71
guidelines, Internet resources, 217–218

H

hazard ratio, definition, 197
HbA1c point-of-care testing scenarios
critical appraisal process in, 138–142
evaluating in different care settings, 36–37
outcome study, 212
setting questions, 78
treatment decisions and, 71
healthcare management, EBM and, 9
Herceptin, prescribing decision questions, 70
heterogeneity, definition, 197

I

inappropriate reference test bias, definition, 198
inappropriateness, of tests, 17
incidence, definition, 198
inclusion criteria, definition, 198
incorporation bias, definition, 198
index test, definition, 198
indexing bias, definition, 198
inflammatory bowel disease, 70–71
information
need for, 17
sources of, 17, 217–218
value of, 6
INR monitoring, 79
intention-to-treat analysis, 140, 198
internal validity, 150
internal validity criteria, definition, 198
International Federation of Clinical Chemistry web address, 214
Internet
access to, 101
sources of evidence, 217
sources of guidelines, 217–218
statistics sites, 216
Internet websites, 213–218
interventions
evidence application and, 149
in the PICO acronym, 8

K

keywords, selection of, 97–98
knowledge, performance and, 17

L

laboratory handbooks, 17
laboratory information systems, 17, 18
laboratory investigations. *See also* research; study designs
  contributions of, 19
  regulation of, 18
  translation into practice, 18
laboratory medicine, good practice, 15
laboratory tests
  appropriate use of, 10–11, 17
  comparative performance questions, 129–137
  discontinuation of, 30–31
  effectiveness of, 16
  interpretation of, 25–26
  introduction of, 27
  likelihood ratios, 198–200, 207–209
  predictive values, 199, 201, 206
  recommendation of, 19
  relationship with disease, 10
  sensitivity, 94*f*, 203, 206
  specificity, 94*f*, 203, 206
  use of, clinician questions on, 25, 26
  utility of, 18
  utilization hierarchy, 149*f*
  validity of, 150, 151
  waiting times and, 78–79
language bias, definition, 198
learning log, 181
lifelong learning, 177–181
lifestyle, as confounder, 122
likelihood ratio, 49, 198–200, 207–209
literature reviews
  comprehensive, 144
  question formulation and, 48
longitudinal studies, 230

M

Medical Subject Headings. *See* MeSH terms
MEDION, 96*t*
MEDLINE (PubMed), 95*t*, 101–108. *See also* PubMed
MeSH terms, 97–98, 113*f*
meta-analysis, 93–94, 199
method performance
  levels of, 29
  mode of care and, 29–30
  outcomes related to, 28–29
methodological quality, 127–128
modes of care, changes, 29–30
Moses-type SROC curves. *See* SROC

N

n-of-1 trials, 199
National Academy of Clinical Biochemistry (NACB), 138
National Institute for Clinical Excellence (NICE), 214
negative likelihood ratio, 199, 207
negative predictive value (NPV), 199, 206, 234, 237
normal (result), definition, 199
null hypothesis, statement of, 211
number needed to harm (NNH), 199
number needed to treat (NNT), 200

O

observational study, definition, 200. *See also* cohort studies
observer bias, definition, 200
odds, definition, 200, 201
odds ratio, 123*f*, 196, 200, 208
operational outcomes
  change management and, 152–153
  of changes in practice, 163
  definition, 13–14
  measures of, 13–14
  question formulation, 78–81
operator bias, definition, 200
outcome. *See also* results
  assessment of, 19
  CASP checklist for, 246–248
  clinical, 13
  consistency of, 137
  diagnostic accuracy and, 62
  economic, 14, 27–28, 74, 82–88, 159–160, 164
  evidence application and, 149
  impact of critical appraisal on, 249–254
  measurement of, 135, 153, 160, 164
  method performance and, 28–29
  operational, 13–14, 78–81, 152–153, 163
  patient well-being and, 142, 150
  in the PICO acronym, 8
  process-related, 14*t*
  test access and, 12
  test effectiveness and, 16
  test timing issues, 66
  test utilization and, 10, 149*f*
  viewpoints on, 145

P

p values, reporting of, 141
partial verification bias, definition, 200
patient management
  changes to, 142, 159–160
  decision making in, 133
  test utility and, 19, 150
patient values
  change in practice and, 159
  decision making and, 6–7
  test acceptance and, 163
patients. *See also* confounder variables
  impact of care on, 12
  in the PICO acronym, 8, 49, 54–85, 122, 149, 151, 157–164
  relationships with doctors, 45–48
performance bias, definition, 200
performance reviews, 182–186
PICCO, 51–53
PICO principle
  application of, 12
  audit of performance, 180–183
  components of, 49–53
  definition, 200
  evidence application and, 149
  in evidence selection, 122–125
  question formulation and, 8, 49–88
  in the search process, 97
point-of-care testing (POCT)
  analytical performance questions, 74–75
  cases for change to, 29–30
  for *Chlamydia*, 83–84
  critical appraisal process in, 138–142
  economic outcomes and, 82–83
  evaluating modes of care, 36–37
  HbA1c scenarios, 3, 37–37, 71, 78, 138–142, 212
  outcome study, 212
  setting questions, 78
policymaking
  evidence-based medicine and, 9
  screening programs and, 28
populations
  applicability of, 132, 137, 141, 151, 157, 161
  evidence application and, 149
  in the PICO acronym, 8, 54–85, 96, 122
positive likelihood ratio, 200, 207
positive predictive value (PPV)
  calculation of, 206, 234, 237
  definition, 201
post-test odds, definition, 201
post-test probability, definition, 201
power calculation
  definition, 201
  examples, 210–212
  reporting of, 141
  sample size and, 212
pre-test odds, definition, 201
pre-test probability, definition, 201
precision
  reporting of, 141
  study description of, 161
  of study results, 158
  validation of, 151
predictions, question formulation, 66–73
prevalence, definition, 54–57, 201
primary research
  conduct of, 122*f*
  critical appraisal of, 124
  description, 93
prior tests, 49
process assessments, evidence in, 32
process outcomes, surrogate measures of, 14*t*
professional associations, 86, 214
prognosis
  definition, 201
  question formulation, 66–73
  study design choice, 92*t*
prognostic study design, 92*t*, 235
prognostic tests, CASP checklist, 242–245
prostate cancer, 59–60, 210–212
prostate-specific antigen scenarios, 55–56, 75–76
protocols, adherence to, 131, 141
Public Health Resource Unit (PHRU) web address, 214
publication bias, definition, 201
PubMed
  article delivery, 110–111
  Boolean commands, 100*t*
  Boolean search operators, 108
  "Clinical Queries" option, 101, 102*f*, 106, 107*f*, 109*f*
  description, 95, 95*t*
  features, 101–108
  "Limits" parameters, 103*f*, 105*f*
  "Limits" tab, 101, 102*f*
  MeSH option, 98, 113*f*
  "Related Articles" option, 111*f*
  screen shots, 101*f*–107*f*, 109*f*–111*f*, 113*f*–114*f*
  search results, 104*f*, 106*f*, 107*f*, 110*f*, 114*f*
  web address, 213
pulmonary emboli, 103–111

Q

QUADAS checklist, 126*t*, 201, 214
questions
approach to, 91
context of, 45–48
definition, 8
focused, 144
formulation of, 8–9, 24–32, 48, 62–65
levels of evidence and, 238
PICO and, 49–88
problems and, 45
for sample searches, 96–99
structure of, 24
study designs and, 92*t*, 230–236
types of, 97

R

race, as confounder, 122
RAMMbo acronym, 127–128
allocation aspect, 127, 131, 132, 135
blinding aspect, 127, 130, 140
definition, 201
maintenance aspect, 127
measurement aspect, 127, 131
outcomes aspect, 127
recruitment aspect, 131, 134
study methods, 128*t*
random effects model, definition, 202
randomization, definition, 202
randomized controlled trial (RCT)
critical appraisal of, 124
definition, 202
design of, 231
questions answered by, 92*t*, 231
receiver operating characteristic (ROC) curves, 131, 202–203
reference ranges, 151, 157, 161
reference standard, 130, 131, 202
relative benefit increase, definition, 202
relative risk, definition, 202
relative risk reduction, definition, 202
research. *See also* study designs
primary research, 93, 122*f*, 124
relevance of, 122
secondary, 93–94, 124
types of, 93–94
resource allocation
appraisal of, 142
change in practice and, 160
test selection and, 132
waiting time reduction and, 82–83
resources, Internet, 213–218
results. *See also* outcome
interpretation of, 17
reporting of, 141, 145
reticulocyte hemoglobin tests, 63
review bias, 131, 202
risk analysis
change management and, 159
Down syndrome screening, 75
for screening programs, 163
study design choice, 92*t*
test use and, 10
risk factors for disease, 54–57, 92*t*
risk ratio (RR), definition, 202
ROC (receiver operating characteristics), 131, 202–203

S

sample sizes, statistical power and, 137, 141, 210–211, 212
ScHARR web site, 215
screening programs
application of evidence to, 160–164
Chlamydia, 82
for colon neoplasia, 58–59
Down syndrome, 75
evaluation of test effectiveness, 39–40
policymaking and, 28
for prostate cancer, 59–60
question formulation, 58–61
search process
audit of performance, 184
clinical questions and, 95
narrowing terms used, 99
question formulation, 96–99
search types, 97
steps in, 97
secondary research, 93, 124
selection bias
cohort design and, 134
definition, 203
self-test, 258–259
sensitivity, diagnostic
calculation of, 206, 234, 237
definition, 203
illustration, 94*f*
power calculations and, 210
reporting of, 132

setting issues
Chlamydia screening, 82
INR monitoring, 79
outcomes and, 78
PICO and (PICOS), 49–50
study applicability and, 157, 161
urinary tract infection tests, 62
significance, statistical, 212
SnNout, definition, 203
socioeconomic status, as confounder, 122
specificity, diagnostic
calculation of, 206
definition, 203
illustration, 94*f*
reporting of, 132
spectrum bias
definition, 203
description, 121
identification of, 131, 132
SpPin, definition, 203
SROC (Summary Receiver Operating Characteristic), 204
STARD
acronym, 204
website, 215
statistical tools, appraisal of, 141
STEP checklist, 126*t*, 204
study designs
appropriateness of, 229–237
assessing quality of, 123
avoiding confounders, 122–123
comparator test method, 158
question formulation and, 48, 92*t*, 99, 230–236
relevance of, 134
result reporting, 136
sample sizes, 137
systematic review
creation of, 18
critical appraisal process, 124, 143–145
definition, 205
description, 93
reliability of, 121

T

target condition, definition, 205
test acceptance and, 164
test request orders, 12*f*, 17, 18
The Clinical Biochemist Reviews, 213
therapy questions, 92*t*
time management, 17
timing issues
PICO principle and (PICOT), 50
prognostic tests and, 66
treatment selection and, 70
waiting times and, 78–79
treatment selection. *See also* decision making
Chlamydia screening and, 79–80
question formulation, 70–73
study design choice, 92*t*
TRIP (Turning Research into Practice) database, 96*t*
troponin scenarios
analytical performance questions, 74–75
prognostic performance, 66
question formulation, 54

U

urinary tract infections, 62
utility of tests, investigation of, 18
utilization
audits of, 30, 178, 188, 194
hierarchy for tests, 149*f*

V

validity. *See also* external validity; internal validity
comparator test method, 158, 162
definition, 205
of study results, 158
of tests, 150
value-for-money (VFM) requirements, 153*f*
verification bias, 131, 196, 200

W

Web of Science, 95*t*
websites, useful, 213–218